D0454822

American River College Library
4700 College Oak Drive
Sacramento, CA 95841

Aging and Ethnicity

Knowledge and Services

Second Edition

Donald E. Gelfand, Ph.D. is Professor and former Chair of the Department of Sociology at Wayne State University. His interests span both basic and applied areas of aging. He has conducted research on the relationship of ethnicity to aging among Salvadorans, African Americans, Russian Jews and a number of other White ethnic groups. Since joining the faculty at Wayne State University in 1991, he has been involved in research on long-term care issues among Native Americans and attitudes toward cancer and cancer treatment among African Americans and Latinos. His current activities focus on end-of-life issues. He is Coordinator of the Wayne State University Interdisciplinary End-of-Life Project which includes 34 faculty from 14 different departments across the university. In 1990 he was a Visiting Research Fellow at Australian National University and a Senior Fulbright Fellow in Darmstadt, Germany in 1982. He has served as Associate Director of the National Policy Center on Older Women and as a Senior Research Associate at the National Council on the Aging. His text, *The Aging Network, Program and Services*, 5th edition, was published by Springer Publishing Company in 1999.

Aging and Ethnicity
Knowledge and Services

Second Edition

Donald E. Gelfand, PhD

Copyright © 2003 by Springer Publishing Company, Inc.

All rights reserved

No part of this publication may be reproduced, stored in a retrieval system, or transmitted in any form or by any means, electronic, mechanical, photocopying, recording, or otherwise, without the prior permission of Springer Publishing Company, Inc.

Springer Publishing Company, Inc.
536 Broadway
New York, NY 10012-3955

Acquisitions Editor: Helvi Gold
Production Editor: Janice Stangel
Cover design by Joanne Honigman

03 04 05 06 07 / 5 4 3 2 1

Library of Congress Cataloging-in-Publication Data

Gelfand, Donald E.
  Aging and ethnicity : knowledge and services / Donald E. Gelfand. — 2nd ed.
    p. cm.
  Includes bibliographical references and index.
  ISBN 0-8261-7421-3
    1. Minority aged—United States. 2. Minority aged—Services for—United
States. I. Title.
  HQ1064.U5G378 2003
  305.26'0973—dc22   2003057355

Printed in the United States of America by Maple-Vail Book Manufacturing Group.

To Katharine,
for her love and support

Contents

Preface

As the new century progresses, and for the foreseeable future, issues of ethnicity are going to remain important. Any belief that the role of ethnicity in modern life would be eliminated was dispelled by events of the 1990s, in such disparate places as Serbia and Rwanda. We cannot afford to understand world events without understanding the role of ethnicity in people's lives.

The new edition of *Aging and Ethnicity* has been developed from this perspective. I have devoted greater attention to the impact of immigration on the United States and have been able to utilize data about important ethnic groups that was becoming available from the 2000 census as this edition was being prepared. I have also tried to grapple with the development of a model that would be helpful to providers working with older persons from diverse ethnic backgrounds. Unfortunately, because of a lack of adequate new data about groups from European backgrounds, some sections on these populations have been eliminated. Where possible, however, comparisons are drawn between older persons from these ethnic backgrounds and individuals whose ethnic origins have different roots.

As was true of my first effort, this edition is not intended to serve as a comprehensive review of all of the literature and research now available on aging and ethnicity. Instead, I have tried to pull together the issues and themes that I believe are important to understanding and, hopefully, meeting the needs of older people from diverse backgrounds and enhancing the knowledge of practitioners attempting to address those needs.

Introduction

Ethnicity has long been an important concept in sociology. The large influxes of immigrants in the United States during the early 1900s coincided with the development of sociology as a discipline in the United States. Sociologists of the Chicago school, as well as reporters such as Jacob Riis, were concerned about the immigrants living in squalid conditions in poor neighborhoods. Their penultimate question was about the ability of many of these groups to assimilate and become part of the melting pot of American society. During the 1900s, ethnicity could be examined in terms of what seemed to be unchangeable racial designations: White, Negro, American Indian, Oriental.

Sociological analyses of ethnicity are now much more difficult. Sociologists and cultural commentators formerly examined the major white ethnic groups and contrasted these groups with so-called minority populations comprised of major non-White racial groups in the United States. These populations included Blacks, Hispanics, Asians, and American Indians. In recent years, terminology has changed, but not the important alteration in American ethnic patterns, in which, as the 1990 and 2000 censuses indicate, the diversity of the American population is increasing dramatically. What is important about this diversity is not only its size, but the origin of many of the groups, the socioeconomic background and circumstances under which many of the new Americans arrive and live in the United States, and the blurring of distinct ethnic identities. These issues are examined in Chapter 2. However, there are changes in American society unrelated to ethnicity, which add to the complexity of the current situation. These changes need to be discussed, in order to set the stage for a discussion of aging and ethnicity.

GROWTH OF THE OLDER POPULATION

Population growth is the result of either natural increase, which occurs because of a surplus of births over deaths, or immigration. A large population in a country usually means that the population will also grow through natural increase, that is, birth of children. The rate of increase is dependent on the fertility rate of the population, that is, the number of children born to each woman. A high fertility rate is needed to maintain the size of a population, if there is a large older group. Countries with a low fertility rate and a large older population may begin to see a reduction in the total population in the country. This trend is already evident in Japan and Germany. Not only does the population decrease, but the ratio of older people to younger people can create strains on the social welfare system. This is most evident in pension systems based on the model in which workers pay into a program that then provides benefits to retirees.

In the United States, this type of debate has been centered on the viability of the Social Security system. Since Social Security is a pay-as-you-go system that depends on the contributions of workers to finance the benefits of retirees, a significant drop in the number of workers and a growth in the number of retirees creates problems in continuing the benefits. When Social Security was enacted in 1935, there were approximately 13 workers for every retiree. In 2000, there were estimated to be only two workers for each retiree (Palen, 2001).

The situation facing the United States and other industrialized countries can be seen by comparison with countries such as Mexico. In Mexico, there is a clear population pyramid, with the largest number of individuals below the age 4 years and decreasing numbers of individuals at each succeeding age (Figure 1).

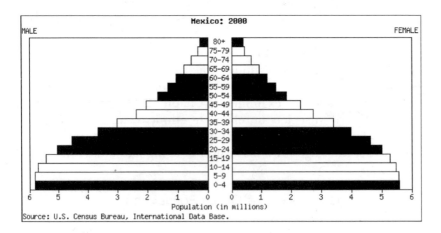

FIGURE 1   Population distribution by age in Mexico: 2000.

A similar population pyramid would be found in many developing countries. Compared to the population pyramid analogy, the population in the United States in the year 2000 already appeared to be more of a rectangle (Figure 2). In 2025 (Figure 3), the U.S. population clearly will no longer even approximate a pyramidal shape. There will be bulges in the 30–44 and 60–64 age categories. Rather than a steady narrowing

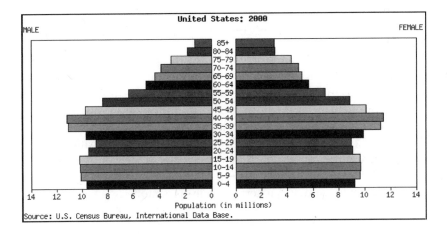

FIGURE 2   Population distribution by age of U.S. population.

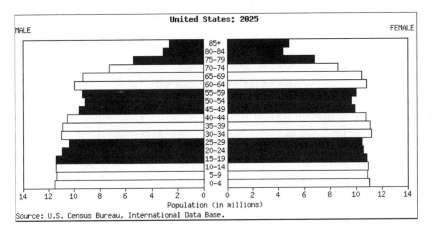

FIGURE 3   Population distribution by age of U.S. population: 2025.

of the population as age increases, there is a bulge at the middle age ranges. As this group continues to age, the bulge at the middle age will move up into a continued flattening of the shape of the pyramid into a rectangle.

The growth of the older population is projected to accelerate after about 2015. During the 15 years prior to this date, the growth of the population over the age of 65 is projected to be much slower than it was during the 1900s. This slow growth rate stems from the lack of growth among the 65–74 age cohort (U.S. Census Bureau, 2001). This slow growth is a result of lower fertility in the United States during the Great Depression.

The changes in the age distribution of the population found in the United States can also be found in other countries. In Australia, for example, the population over the age of 65 is expected to be 17% of the total population by 2020. In Japan, the population over the age of 65 is expected to reach a staggering 27% of the population by the year 2020 (Commonwealth of Australia, 2000). The implications of this change are significant in their impact on many aspects of life, including family relationships, the role older persons have in society, and their impact on health and social service delivery systems.

LIFE EXPECTANCY

The increased proportion of older persons in the general population is naturally related to the fantastic increase in life expectancy that occurred during the twentieth century. The life expectancy of an American child born in 1900 was 46 years. Currently, in the United States, life expectancy for a child born in 2000 is 77.1 years. Although this figure is important, it does not provide us with information about the cohort of individuals who will be classified as elderly during the next 50 years. Some more relevant data is shown in Table 1, which projects the older American population by age through the year 2050.

This table utilizes a moderately conservative estimate of population growth. The projection does not take into account any major breakthroughs in heart disease or cancer, the two most common causes of death. It also does not take into account any negative impacts on population growth, such as a major war, new biological problems, or the catastrophic effects of illnesses such as the AIDS.

Unfortunately, life expectancy still varies among ethnic populations. Even with the disparities in life expectancy among ethnic groups, the numbers of older people in each of these groups will be growing dramatically in the twenty-first century. The proportion of older people in the

TABLE 1   Older Population by Age: 2000 to 2050 (%)

Year and census date	Age in years			
	65–74	75–84	85 and over	65 and over
2000	6.7	4.5	1.6	12.8
2010	7	4.4	2	13.3
2020	9.5	4.7	2.1	16.4
2030	10.9	6.7	2.5	20.1
2040	9.1	7.9	3.7	20.7
2050	8.8	6.8	4.8	20.4

Source: Administration on Aging, n.d.

population of each of these groups may also grow, if groups that have typically had large numbers of children begin to reduce their family size.

Even with this conservative estimate of population growth among the total U.S. population, clearly, all segments of the older population will grow significantly. Most important, however, is the large increase in the older cohorts of the older population. If we employ the now-conventional distinction of the "young old" (ages 65 to 74), "old old" (ages 75 to 84), and "oldest of the old" (age 85 and above), the oldest of the old are obviously a rapidly increasing group. The percentage will be more than double the 1.6% of 2000 by the year 2040, and will continue to grow. The approximately 5 million women and more than 2 million men age 85 and over, in 2025 (U.S. Census Bureau, n.d.), may place major demands on family members and health and social services. Families and providers will have to meet the challenges of (1) financial security, (2) provision of adequate medical care for a group with substantial medical needs, and (3) provision of a variety of services to a group whose ability to carry out important activities of daily living may be limited.

All individuals have an idea of the type of lifestyle they would like to maintain or attain as they grow older. These goals may vary among ethnic groups and involve long-standing cultural traditions, socioeconomic status, and possible acculturation to norms and beliefs that are considered "American." Understanding and helping older members of diverse ethnic groups meet these goals is a large agenda.

CHANGING LIVING PATTERNS

At the end of World War II, Americans in large numbers took advantage of the opportunities provided by low-rate mortgages and moved en masse to the suburbs. American soldiers returning from the war enrolled in colleges with tuition support from the GI Bill. Women forced out of factories, because of the return of the soldiers, joined their husbands in new suburban homes and raised the generation of children that we now term the "baby boom" generation. The vast majority of these individuals have remained in suburban communities as they grew older and thus fit the patterns of "aging in place." Their adult children, however, may have moved to other communities around the country.

At the end of the twentieth century, the impact of these events became apparent. Instead of a population of older individuals living in densely populated neighborhoods in central cities, the older population is now predominantly a suburbanized group. In many cities, ethnic neighborhoods, with such names as Little Italy or Polonia, are either completely gone or shells of their former self. Ethnic restaurants may remain, as attractions for tourists, but the ethnic populations have now dispersed to suburban areas, where density is much lower. Many of the urban ethnic communities that continue to exist in inner cities can be characterized as poor minority communities.

The suburbanization of the population, and the dispersal of younger family members to communities around the country, create a variety of problems for families with older members who are in need of assistance.

ORGANIZATION

This volume is dedicated to the ethnic elderly living in the United States. Chapter 1 begins with an overview of some of the theories of aging, and the meaning of the seemingly elusive concept of *ethnicity*. The major concentration is on the possible types of allegiance of older persons to ethnic identity, and the positive or negative impacts of ethnicity on older persons. The reasons for some of the gaps in knowledge are examined in a brief review of the problems of conducting research on ethnicity and aging.

Chapter 2 is a detailed look at immigration—one of the major factors in the current age distribution of the ethnic aged. Immigration is also a major factor in the growth of the American population, and in the ethnic diversity of communities throughout the country.

The history and current situation of the ethnic aged is presented in Chapter 3. Because of a lack of adequate data on groups from European backgrounds, attention in this chapter focuses on minority elderly: African Americans, Asians, Latinos, and Native Americans. The socioeconomic backgrounds and health and mental health statuses of each of these groups are the primary concerns of the chapter.

All individuals face challenges as they grow older. One of these challenges includes maintaining a stable environment that provides a sense of security. Chapter 4 examines the differences among the ethnic elderly that affect their sense of security and the ways in which various ethnic and racial groups strive to attain this sense of security.

No topic has been more widely discussed in recent years than the role of the family in the lives of older people. Particular emphasis has been placed on the role of family members as providers of assistance. Chapter 5 focuses on differences in the assistance provided to the ethnic aged by family members, and the factors that play a part in these family patterns. Chapter 5 also discusses the role of religious organizations and religion in the lives of the ethnic aged. Although religions affiliation is a forbidden question on the U.S. Census, there is little doubt that religion and spirituality are vital elements in the lives of many older people.

The first five chapters lay the groundwork for an examination of service delivery issues that have an impact on the lives of the ethnic aged. An analytic model for these issues is offered in Chapter 6, and factors that may determine the use of services by the ethnic aged are explored. Special attention is paid to the problems of effective outreach, with examples drawn from health-related topics.

Chapter 7 examines individual programs and services that are currently available to older people. The focus is not on a detailed explanation of each of these programs and services, but rather on how they could incorporate elements that would address concerns and values of the ethnic aged. Programs and services specifically oriented to older people are first discussed, followed by health and mental health services that provide primary and secondary prevention.

The concluding chapter is an effort to consider steps needed to develop more knowledge about the ethnic aged and provide them with the assistance they need. Three topics are examined: (1) assumptions that have been part of the paradigms of research and services delivery in the area of ethnicity and aging, (2) revised assumptions that can be used in research and service development for the ethnic aged, and (3) a model to assess the factors that are important in providing effective services to men and women from diverse ethnic backgrounds.

The terms *African American, Latinos,* and *Native American* have been used throughout the book to designate major American minority groups. In order to be consistent with current data collection sources, the terms *Black* will also be used at times, instead of *African American,* and *Hispanic* rather than *Latino.*

REFERENCES

Administration on Aging. (n.d.). *Older population by age: 1900 to 2050.* Retrieved August 26, 2002, from *http://www.aoa.dhhs.gov/aoa/STATS/AgePop2050.html*

Commonwealth of Australia. (2000). *Australia, Japan: A comparison of aged care in Australia and Japan.* Canberra: Author.

Palen, J. (2001). *Social problems for the twenty-first century.* New York: McGraw-Hill.

U.S. Census Bureau. (n.d.). *Projections of the total resident population by 5 year age group and sex with special age categories: 2025–2045.* Retrieved August 26, 2002, from: *http://www.census.gov/population/projections/national/summary/np-t3-f..txt*

U.S. Census Bureau. (2001). *The 65 years and over population: 2000.* Retrieved April 22, 2002, from *http://www.census.gov/prod/2001/pubs/c2kbr01-10.pdf*

U.S. Census Bureau, International Database. (n.d.). Retrieved June 1, 2002, from *http://www.census.gov/ipc/www.idpyr.html*

Chapter One

Ethnicity, Gerontological Theory, and Research

ETHNICITY AND THEORIES OF AGING

The field of aging, or gerontology, is a relatively new one. Many of its first investigators and practitioners saw a need to formulate a distinct theoretical model. Although significant theoretical development has occurred in gerontology since the end of World War II, attention to the role of ethnicity and race in the aging process has been limited.

Disengagement Theory

The first major theoretical approaches in gerontology stemmed from functionalist sociology. Research conducted by the University of Chicago resulted in the formulation of *disengagement theory*, which, briefly stated, postulates that all people disengage from society as they become older. This disengagement is intrinsic to the aging process, because older people need to develop equilibrium in their lives as they go through life's final stages. The older individual also needs to prepare for death. In terms of ethnic background, a number of questions can be asked:

1. Do individuals from different ethnic backgrounds disengage at the same time in their lives and in the same manner?
2. Does their disengagement include disengagement from any involvement in activities related to their ethnic background?

3. Does their disengagement include disengagement from ethnic values and behaviors that are normative in the ethnic culture?

Unfortunately, these questions have never been asked or answered. Disengagement theory has also failed to maintain its place as an important theory in the field. As Hochschild (1975) pointed out, the demise of disengagement theory results from a number of flaws in its theoretical structure, including its lack of testability. Because of this, the formulators of disengagement theory were forced to label individuals who did not disengage as "failed disengagers," rather than as individuals able to develop an alternative approach to growing older.

Activity Theory

The same testability problem afflicts disengagement theory's rival, *activity theory*. A person who does not disengage as they grow older may become involved with a variety of activities that are available when they are no longer employed. Activity theorists argue that older individuals who are involved in a variety of activities are more successful in their aging. The primary question that could be asked here is: Are older persons involved with activities relating to their ethnic background more successful in their aging? An answer to this question is difficult, because of the controversy associated with the concept of successful aging. A more appropriate and answerable question is: Does adherence to ethnic values, norms, and behaviors relate positively to older persons' satisfaction with their life and to their mental health?

Continuity Theory

Continuity theory allows flexibility in viewing different individuals' lifestyles. Rather than seeing later years as separate from other stages of life, continuity theory examines older persons' behaviors as they relate to their whole life course. What would be most valued by some individuals in later years may not be valued by others, because these same things have not been valued at earlier periods. In this sense, aging is seen as a continuation of earlier stages of the individual's life, rather than as a separate and unique period.

The later years certainly have issues that are specific to this stage of life, but there are also unique issues in adolescence, early adulthood, and middle-age. The repertoire of values and behaviors that an individual develops at an earlier age will be used to meet the issues of aging. If values and behaviors stemming from a particular ethnic culture are part of this repertoire, then it is likely that the individual will turn to them to meet some of the physical changes, role changes, and bereavement issues that occur in later years. Although the utilization of ethnic values may be discontinuous with their past, it may represent a determination by older persons to shape their later years differently from their earlier ones.

Role and Exchange Theory

A final reason for tapping into lost or unused ethnic values and behaviors can be seen from the perspective of two additional theoretical perspectives in gerontology: *role theory* and *exchange theory*. As is true of continuity theory, both of these theoretical approaches are common in general social-psychological and sociological theory. The basic question for role theory is, What roles are available for individuals who occupy different statuses? For the older person, it has often been said that there are no roles available, unless a role of disengager is accepted as valid. In this sense, aging was termed the "roleless role." Theorists such as Cowgill (1988) would argue that this lack of roles is most common in industrialized, urbanized societies. There may be roles for the older person, however, within specific ethnic groups. This availability of roles may encourage the older person to become more involved in ethnic cultures.

In the larger society, the experience of the older person may not be seen as having much intrinsic value. Within an ethnic culture, the older person may find that they are esteemed because of their experience and their greater knowledge of ethnic lore and history. The older person can exchange this knowledge for a position of deferment and respect from younger individuals. In some ethnic cultures, there are thus distinct advantages for the older person.

STRUCTURAL AND ATTITUDINAL CHANGE

This brief overview of some theoretical approaches in aging illustrates how the variability of ethnicity can be incorporated into theoretical models. However, observing societal changes that provide support for theoretical models is not always easy. There may seem to be no changes occurring within a society, unless investigators are thorough in their efforts. Kendig's (1988) research on changes in attitudes and care for the elderly in Japan clearly points this out. Examining caregiving patterns, Kendig finds that values about the elderly and assistance have not changed among younger generations, but that the structures and actual caregiving arrangements have altered dramatically.

Structural change may occur before attitudinal change—a fact that many civil rights advocates learned during the 1960s, as they attempted to end discrimination against Blacks. Despite 24-hour closed door confrontations between Blacks and Whites, prejudicial attitudes resisted change. Legislative changes that required desegregation were found to be more effective in producing change. Even though the White worker in the factory did not alter his prejudicial feelings toward his new Black coworker, he accepted the Black worker, once desegregation was mandated (Reitzes, 1959).

In the same manner, Greek women may profess a continued desire to provide care for their older parents, even though employment outside the home, the lack of available support from other siblings, and the demands of their immediate family may make the use of formal services a necessity (McCallum & Gelfand, 1990). The extent to which traditional ethnic attitudes remain strong, while specific changes take place in the behaviors of the elderly themselves, their families, and the larger ethnic group, is a major topic for research.

Definitional Components

In order to be consistent in the discussion of ethnicity and aging, some attention must be devoted to the definition of *ethnicity*. Definitions of ethnicity have three major components: (1) the identification of the group as an ethnic or racial group by others, (2) the identification of the group as ethnic or racial by the group members themselves, and (3) specific behavior patterns that distinguish the group. Probably the most well-known definition is that put forth by Gordon (1964), who argued that an ethnic group is one with a sense of peoplehood, based on race, religion, or national origin. Holzberg provides a more detailed discussion:

> Ethnicity, that is, social differentiation based on such cultural criteria as a sense of peoplehood, shared history, a common place of origin, language, dress and free preferences, and participation in particular clubs or voluntary associations, engenders a sense of exclusiveness and self-awareness that one is a member of a distinct and bounded social group. But it is not the ethnic content (markers) per se that constitutes the diacritica of social differentiation. More important for the purposes of social distance are the feelings of

shared particularity, self-identification, and membership in ethnic-exclusive associations. (1982, p. 252)

Ethnicity is shaped "both by agency and structure" (Erdmans, 1995, p. 177). For Whites, being identified as a member of an ethnic group is a matter of choice (agency), but discrimination and immigration laws may limit or make this choice impossible for people of color.

Because racial background is only one of the dimensions, racial and ethnic groups are not distinct entities. Racial groups are one distinct type of group whose ethnic identity is based on their physical characteristics. A group may be identified as a race by its members or by others (Alba, 1992). Racial categories are thus socially constructed.

Past efforts to classify individuals as members of one of three races are now seen to have little basis in reality, because of the diversity of the gene pool around the world. As Berlin (1998) notes, race is also historically constructed, and racial designations can change over time. An example is the designation of Mexicans by the U.S. census. The 1920 census designated Mexicans as "Whites." In 1930, Mexicans were now placed in a separate racial category. In 1950, Mexicans were again classified as Whites, but current census usage places Mexicans among the separate category of "Hispanics" (Rodriguez, 2001).

Even if "White," "Black," "Hispanic," and "Native American" are used to classify the ethnic/racial backgrounds of individuals, the continued growth in intermarriage rates in the United States creates problems. Overall, intermarriages among ethnic/racial groups are now estimated to have grown to 3 million, from 500,000 in 1970 (Pugh, 2001). The majority of these intermarriages are among groups from European backgrounds (*American Culture*, n.d.). During the 1990s, many individuals were checking the choice of "Other" on surveys that asked racial background, because of their mixed ethnic and racial backgrounds. The multiethnic background of professional golfer Tiger Woods became a symbol of the ethnic complexity of the United States. In response to concerns that a significant amount of important information about ethnicity was being lost, the 2000 U.S. census allowed multiple choices of ethnic identity. The result was that 2% of the American population identified themselves as being from more than one racial group (Schmitt, 2001). Officials at the Census Bureau believe that, if a category of "Other" had not been included, the number of individuals choosing multiple categories would have been greater. The four most common multiracial choices categories were "White and Black," "White and Asian," "White and American Indian," and "White and some other race." The overall 2000 census data will now be presented in 63 racial categories. In 1990, there were only 5 racial categories in the census.

Nationhood and Ethnicity

As events in the early 1990s indicated, national identity, ethnicity, and nationhood are not necessarily defined in similar ways. One definition of ethnicity places its emphasis on a shared historical past of a group (Schermerhorn, 1970). In Eastern Europe, areas such as Lithuania and Latvia have not had nationhood since World War II. The sense of national identity based on ethnic background remained in these communities, despite their incorporation into the former Soviet Union. In Yugoslavia, nationhood was established after World War II but national identity never took root. Instead, long-standing ethnic identity remained constant in the lives of Serbs, Croats, Macedonians, Bosnians, and Montenegrians. In Canada, the desire for recognition of ethnic identity among French Canadians has resulted in secessionist movements that have waxed and waned. In Spain, Basques have never given up their fight for separation.

The most frequent discussion of ethnicity focuses around groups that live in a society that includes other ethnic groups. The dissolution of the Soviet Union and Yugoslavia in the 1990s represents a period in which ethnic groups reasserted their right to be self-governing entities based on a distinct sense of peoplehood, history, and attachment to a particular geographic area.

Ethnicity and ethnic groups precede the concept of nationhood in historical context. Many modern nations have failed to bring diverse ethnic groups with varying norms and cultures into a national framework. In some cases, historical events made the boundaries of particular nations logical. In other cases, national borders were arbitrarily shaped, with enormous consequences. This is particularly true in Africa, where nations were developed out of former European colonies. Little regard was paid to the historical backgrounds, cultures, and hostilities of existing tribes. Interethnic warfare and conflict has been one unfortunate feature of modern African countries.

Ethnic Groups and Minority Groups

The processes that pertain to ethnic groups also affect groups considered to be "minority." However, important issues differentiate minority groups in particular from ethnic groups in general. The sociologist Louis Wirth provided the classic definition of a minority:

> We may define a minority as a group of people who, because of their physical or cultural characteristics are singled out from the others in the society in

which they live for differential and unequal treatment, and who therefore regard themselves as objects of collective discrimination. The existence of a minority in a society implies the existence of a dominant group with higher social status and greater privileges. Minority status carries with it the exclusion from full participation in the life of the society. (1945, p. 348)

There are a number of key elements in this definition. First is the discrimination against ethnic group members because of their characteristics. Second, the ethnic group members perceive themselves as being the objects of discrimination because of their inferior position. Makielski (1973) classifies discrimination against minorities in terms of the different types of deprivation they suffer, which include legal, economic, social, and subjective deprivation. Legal deprivation refers to discrimination based on the lesser legal standing of the group; economic deprivation refers to lower income resulting from poor job opportunities. Social deprivation manifests itself in a number of forms, including the forced residence of all members of the group together, a lack of recognition of achievement, and stereotyping. Subjective deprivation refers to the feeling on the part of the group that they have been, or are being, deprived. This sense of deprivation is often the first aspect of changing the lives of minorities. With their recognition of deprivation, minority groups can begin to organize to change their condition.

The dominant culture may also begin to change as it interacts with minority cultures. African American culture and music have been an important part of American life. African American-originated music formed the roots of rock and roll. African American speech patterns have also influenced American English.

There is a gap in the United States between sociological definition of a minority group and the administrative designation of specific ethnic/racial groups as minorities. Glazer and Moynihan (1970) argued that ethnic groups can be seen as interest groups. As such, some ethnic groups have been able to have themselves designated as a minority, but others lack this important designation. Currently, a major example of this gap is the lack of any official designation of the large, growing, and diverse Arab population in the United States as a minority, despite the fact that this group meets many of the criteria in Wirth's definition.

In the United States, official recognition of minority status results in a group becoming eligible for a variety of special programs and benefits, ranging from affirmative action to minority set-asides in federal contracts. Although only people of color—African Americans, Latinos, Asians, and Native Americans—have been accorded this title, other groups, such as gays and lesbians, meet the Wirth definition and would value the minority designation.

ETHNICITY AND IDENTITY

Examining behavior for signs of ethnic values is a difficult process. One element to look for is a sense of ethnic identity on the part of an individual. This may be expressed by participation in ethnic organizations or by the reading of literature or magazines about the ethnic group. A person may thus join a particular church because of the concentration of people from the same ethnic background. An absence of these types of behaviors does not necessarily mean that the person is devoid of any ethnic identity. Ethnicity may not be expressed overtly. Upon questioning, an individual may express a strong sense of identification with their ethnic background.

At this point, the assessment of ethnic identity begins to become problematic. If the individual does not participate with ethnic groups and organizations or does not express an identification with their ethnic background, does that mean that the ethnic background is no longer important? Advocates of ethnicity would argue that overt participation and identification with ethnic backgrounds are only externalized indicators of important internalized norms. As one writer emphatically asserts, ethnicity, "however ignored or suppressed, comes back to haunt us as we advance in years" (Guttmann, 1986, p. 4). From this perspective, ethnic background, however ignored by the individual in terms of day-to-day life, represents internalized norms and values that are always just below the surface of consciousness. Faced with major changes, or simply the process of aging, these ethnic values will assert themselves.

It is difficult to evaluate claims about the continued or reasserted importance of ethnicity in people's lives. Full acceptance means that it is impossible to say that an individual's ethnic background is not important. In this volume, ethnicity is viewed in terms of expressed attitudes and behaviors, rather than internalized attitudes that are not evident through any overt viewpoints and actions.

If the assumption can be made that ethnicity varies in intensity, from no ethnic identification and participation through complete identification and participation, delineating intermediate degrees of involvement in ethnicity should be possible. For the sake of terseness, involvement in ethnicity is here termed *ethnic allegiance*, which can range from nonexistent to complete, with intermediate steps along the way.

Assessing ethnic allegiance requires understanding of whether an individual has allegiance to either ethnic values, behaviors, or both. Possible results of variations in these allegiances are shown in Figure 1.1.

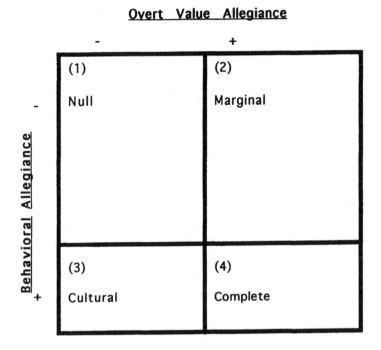

FIGURE 1.1 Degree of ethnic allegiance expressed by individuals.

Null and Complete Allegiance

People who express no overt loyalty to ethnic values, and who exhibit no behaviors that could be considered relevant to their ethnic background, are making clear that they have no allegiance to ethnicity (Cell 1 in Figure 1.1). At the opposite end of the spectrum are individuals who express strong allegiance to ethnic values and who are concerned that their behavior accurately reflects these allegiances. These persons can be considered complete in their allegiance to their ethnic background (Cell 4).

Cultural Allegiance

Many individuals fall into positions that are less consistent and more difficult to characterize. Cell 3 includes persons who do not express allegiance to ethnic values, but who still exhibit behaviors that could be classified as ethnically linked. These behaviors may vary along a complex range. Some individuals and their families maintain a strong interest in the heritage of their ethnic group as represented by its music, dance, theater, and literature. They may also show an interest in the history of the culture and participate in programs related to these cultural legacies. For other persons, the main link to ethnic culture is restricted to eating traditional ethnic foods, which they prepare for their family at home and enjoy in restaurants.

Alba (1985) regards Italian Americans as predominantly cultural in their ethnic allegiance. A study in suburban Baltimore indicated cultural allegiance to ethnicity among a group of middle-class Italian men (Gelfand & Fandetti, 1980). The men's responses indicated an interest in transmitting to their children their pride in Italian culture and history. This could be accomplished through publications and courses. The Italian men would not vote for a politician purely on the basis of Italian background and they expressed no desire to live in a predominantly Italian neighborhood.

In his 1957 book, American Judaism, Nathan Glazer questioned whether Judaism in the United States was not becoming solely related to a "gastric culture," which expressed itself in an interest in bagels and other foods commonly considered Jewish. Similar attitudes have been expressed about the role of food in Italian culture: "If someone doesn't eat pasta, twice a week and on Sunday, he's not Italian" (Johnson, 1985, p. 91). Attendees a ethnic festivals in major American cities may also wonder whether food is not the major factor in many ethnic cultures. Although it is questionable to what extent food can be the most important factor in ethnic cultures, the importance of ethnic foods has often been indicated in studies of the needs and wants of older people. In any case, gastronomic allegiance to ethnic culture places few demands on the individual and the family, and remains basically a nonthreatening type of ethnic affiliation.

Marginal Allegiance

Individuals in Cell 2 express an allegiance to the ethnic values, but their behavior does not indicate a strong allegiance to any particular ethnic background. Terming these individuals "marginal" harkens back to a long-standing sociological concept, which was intended to describe individuals who did not feel comfortable in their ethnic background but also could not join the majority culture.

Lack of allegiance to the values of the ethnic culture might be a factor of choice:

> Indians have spread rather quickly into all levels of the socioeconomic hierarchy. Individuals near the upper end of the socioeconomic scale may have some Indian ancestry, but their lives are not structured by ties to rural Indian communities or by involvement in Indian associations. Indeed, they may not identify themselves as Indians, except under advantageous circumstances, while expressing contempt for, and distancing themselves from less affluent Indians in ghettos and in reservations. (Jarvempa, 1985, p. 36)

The same type of split between their upbringing and their identification has been noted among Hispanics:

> Hispanics having more "successful" integration experiences are more likely to maintain a symbolic connection to their ethnic heritage, as manifested by the continued observance of holidays, the revival of ethnic foods, the practice of cultural rituals, etc. while in the areas of occupation, education, language and residence they are increasingly model Anglos. (Nelson & Tienda, 1985, p. 55)

A person may hide their ethnic background when outside their own ethnic group, in order to avoid discrimination in housing or employment. As media discussions about Native Americans grow, increasing numbers of individuals are acknowledging their Indian heritage. The lack of effort to hide this background indicates it is less harmful, and perhaps even advantageous, to acknowledge a Native American background in the family.

Cells 2 and 3 in Figure 1.1 are the most important elements in the classification of ethnic allegiance, because they reflect a view of ethnicity distinct from the belief that an individual is either an "ethnic" or not. Instead, as is argued throughout this volume, ethnicity can be viewed as an emergent phenomena, one which is created through the interaction between members of a culture with societal conditions and changes. As individuals and families interact with other ethnic groups in the society, their behaviors and values are altered. Behaviors and attitudes, today regarded as marginal, may be the initial steps in reformulation of the ethnic culture. The reformulated culture may contain elements that are retained from the past, as well as elements that are adopted from the host culture. Elements from other ethnic cultures may also be incorporated into the emerging configuration. Formulation and reformulation of ethnic culture is influenced by historical events that specific age cohorts experience. As Erdmans (1995) notes, American

Jewish identity has been affected by industrialization, anti-Semitism, the creation of Israel, and the Arab–Israeli war of 1967.

ETHNIC CULTURE AND CHOICE

Ethnic cultures that survive and flourish are in a constant process of growth and change. A resistance to growth and change may mean the demise of the ethnic culture as it fails to meet the challenges of the environment. These challenges stem from the socioeconomic structure of the society, employment opportunities, political structures, and major value changes.

The Ethnic Matrix

Vasques (1986) labels the complex of norms and values that comprise a culture as the *ethnic matrix*. He argues that this ethnic matrix is "determined by pieces of behavior experienced by each member of the ethnic group, and collectively on a broader scale will be seen as patterns or culture shifts taking place in the group itself" (p. 8).

There are thus a number of possible configurations that could characterize the manifestations of ethnicity and the ethnic culture to which an individual has allegiance. These configurations may be exhibited in a number of attitudinal and behavioral forms selected by the individual. As already noted ethnicity is not only an internalized set of norms, but a set of conscious attitudes that individuals can choose to utilize at various points in their lives. Rather than coming back to haunt them, ethnicity is a means that older people may use to adapt to the process of aging. At various times individuals may utilize their ethnic backgrounds and join ethnic organizations or institutions, because these affiliations provide them emotional or instrumental rewards.

In their study of older widowers in the Philadelphia area, Luborsky and Rubinstein offer examples of this use of ethnicity:

> Mr. Goldberg, aged 73, had been widowed for 3 years. A Jew, he made a distinction between Judaism as an ethnic identity and as a religion. Although hardly religious he had spent much of his life acting on a number of deeply held moral convictions about the need for equality and democracy. He noted that although he was an atheist he felt very much a Jew. Because of his personal concern for social welfare and reform he felt that, although he was not Jewish in a religious sense, he fit well within a Jewish tradition of prophetic protest. He received a large settlement from his wife's insurance policy and

spent a good deal of the money lavishly outfitting a woodworking shop in his basement. His wife was Catholic, and when they married, he reported, he and his wife agreed never to discuss religion in the home. He felt that they had kept to this policy. Mr. Goldberg had three daughters, two of whom 'practice no religion' and one who had become very involved in Judaism.

A year to the day after his wife's death, Mr. Goldberg was wakened by sharp chest pains. Fearing a heart attack, he was hospitalized for tests, which found nothing. Eventually one doctor asked him how he felt toward his deceased wife. He told the doctor of many unresolved feelings: guilt about having treated his wife poorly and fear of estrangement from his daughters. The doctor encouraged him to talk with them about his feelings, which he did.

At one point his religious daughter told him that some of the woodwork in her synagogue needed repair, and she put him in touch with her rabbi. He did the work there and was also able to engage the rabbi in conversations about religion. This represented a reconnection of sorts with Judaism as a religious system. Mr. Goldberg also noted that his wife's death enabled him to appreciate more actively the Jewish religion and cultural tradition. He attributed this change to now being free of the pact with his wife not to discuss religious matters. He also felt that the change had to do with his own aging and an increased concern with his place in the world. (Luborsky & Rubinstein, pp. 38–39)

In contrast to Mr. Goldberg, Mr. Donnell, a 76-year-old Italian, lived in an Italian neighborhood, attended an Italian parish church, and was married to an Italian woman, but had rejected his Italian heritage for many years:

On the other hand, his response to a question about the meaning to him of his Italian identity prompted a vigorous discussion of how the Italians were the "worst" ethnic group, this anchored by several stories of how Italians had caused difficulties for him in several employment situations. The rejection of his heritage was played out in other domains. For example, in his 40s he suffered a mental and physical crisis that among other things led to a psychologically based stomach disorder. He ceased eating Italian foods, which his wife loved to prepare and eat, and substituted bland American foods which he processed in a blender and drank. Additionally, his wife's death, 3 years before the interviews, led to a further redefinition of the life-course situation influencing his ethnic identity. After his wife died, he was able to disentangle himself from his Italian in-laws; for his taste, they were too concerned with being "Italian." He was now quite isolated. This latest synthesis about the meaning of his Italian identity—a pulling away from it—was in fact one in a string of lifelong conflicts and resolutions. His current ethnic feeling was thus influenced by an important life-span event (widowhood) compounded by long-standing conflicts. (Luborsky & Rubinstein, 1987, p. 38)

These men have returned to, or disaffiliated themselves from, their ethnic background, because of some particular life event or life stage that they associate with their Jewish and Italian backgrounds. They have made choices about ethnicity in their own lives. The choices do not need to form an consistent pattern, since there are myriad elements that comprise a particular ethnic culture. At a particular life stage, some of these elements may seem more relevant and others less relevant or too demanding.

The ethnic matrix includes many choices made by the individual about their life. An incomplete list would include choice of type of neighborhood in which to live, choice of spouse, choice of child's name, type of music preferred, ethnic ritual celebrations, use of the "mother tongue," involvement in ethnic politics, or support for bilingual education or ethnic studies (Vasques, 1986). As Vasques recognizes, some of these choices, such as musical preferences, are relatively simple and painless. Other choices, such as the decision to live in a heterogeneous or homogeneous neighborhood, or whether to become involved in ethnic politics, can produce stress. The desire to avoid stress encourages the individual to adopt a marginal approach in which ethnic celebrations are maintained but more demanding ethnic traditions, such as having an older family member live in the home, are disavowed.

Reinvestment of emotional energy and time in the ethnic culture does not mean that the individual is prepared to live in the same manner as their grandparents. A third-generation ethnic person will probably enjoy ethnic cuisine, but adoption of the living patterns or attitudes of the first generation is unlikely. Traditional patterns of ethnic dress and return to residence in an ethnic community are not common among the third generation. The renewal of ethnic loyalties and hostilities in Europe and Africa may also have an impact on the ethnic identification of older Americans. These conflicts focus the vision of many Americans on their ethnic backgrounds. How this focus will affect their interest and involvement in ethnic traditions and values will only be evident over time.

Ethnicity and Religion

The Goldberg and Donnell vignettes include religious elements as major components, and raise the important question of the relationship of religion to ethnicity. Jews in the United States came from many countries. Where Jews have lived for centuries, they have often become important elements of the country's culture. This was certainly true in pre-Nazi era Germany and in earlier periods in Spain. Although Jewish religious practices and ritual provide some common bonds, the attitudes of Jews from Germany, Russia, and Spain may be very different. The same is true among Italian, Irish, and French Catholics. These differences were recognized in this country, where the Catholic Church was allowed to structure local parishes based on the nationality backgrounds of the neighborhood's parishioners. Separating the influence of religion from the discussions of Poles, African Americans, Mexicans, and other groups, omits a major component of ethnic identity among many individuals who belong to these groups. This is also becoming increasingly clear as Americans learn more about the culture of many Arabs from Muslim backgrounds. There are also groups in the United States whose major identity is based on their religious affiliation. Most prominent among these are the Amish and Mormons.

THE POSITIVE IMPACT OF ETHNICITY

Involvement in ethnically related activities is potentially positive in its impact on the aging person. Ethnicity may buffer the older individual against some of the decrements of aging, which encompass physical, social, and emotional facets of a person's life. In Figure 1.2, the possible positive effects of ethnicity are compared to the possible negative effects of age on the individual.

Levelers and Differentiaters

The initial negative aspect of aging in Figure 1.2 (Cell 1) is based on the "age as a leveler" adage, which was current during the early years of the development of gerontology and asserted that, as people get older, all of their prior differences become less important. What becomes most important is that they are all older. Society fails to recognize the differences among older people in temperament, values, norms, and skills, and lumps them together into one negative stereotype of frail, incapable older folks.

Arnold Rose (1965) predicted that society's valuation of age as an overriding determinant of an individual's status would encourage the growth of an aging subculture. In turn, this subculture would become an important force in American society. Fortunately or unfortunately, Rose's prediction was not correct. Part of the reason that the subculture of the aged failed to emerge was the rapid growth of the aged American population. Instead of leading to a subculture based on homogeneity, this increase produced an aged cohort that was diverse and whose

Effects of age	Effects of ethnicity
Age as leveler (1)	Ethnicity as differentiator (2)
Age as negative identity (3)	Ethnicity as positive identity (4)
Age as immutable (5)	Ethnicity as emergent (6)
Age as loss (7)	Ethnicity as gain (8)
Age as forcing adaptation (9)	Ethnicity as means of adaptation (10)

FIGURE 1.2 Comparison of the effects of age and ethnicity.

diversity continues to increase. This diversity includes racial and ethnic diversity (Cell 2) as well as socioeconomic diversity.

As a diverse population, the common interests among older people become muted. This muting, and even disagreement, was clearly evident in the 1989 controversy over the Medicare Catastrophic Health Plan. This important legislation limited the inpatient hospital expenses of older patients, capped their out-of-pocket medical expenses, and represented the first commitment of the Medicare system to reimbursements for prescription drugs. Many affluent elderly resented the payments they would have to make to finance this legislation and effectively pressured Congress for repeal of the legislation, even before it went into effect.

Part of the responsibility for this debacle can be laid at the feet of politicians and specialists in aging who failed to recognize the current diversity in the aging population. Advocates of programs for the aged mistakenly assumed that older people would unanimously support any new legislation beneficial to older Americans as a group.

Age and Ethnicity as Identifiers

Despite this lack of interest in group solidarity, it is unlikely that many older people will reject all of the negative valuations placed by society on the older person (Cell 3). This includes a negative evaluation of physical attributes, mental agility, job performance, and even worthiness as a consumer segment. The older individual whose physical and mental functioning is high is held out as an exception to the normal aging process. These 90-year-old individuals are featured and applauded on talk shows. Despite these appearances, the proliferation of anti-aging formulas and creams makes clear that evidence of getting older is a negative status to be avoided, if at all possible.

In contrast to the negative status accorded aging in most industrialized societies and the lack of positive roles that correspond with this status, ethnicity can be a positive force (Cell 4). Although the image of ethnicity may be romanticized in ethnic festivals that take place around the country, ethnic images are, for the most part, positive. There remain many ways an older person can assert or reassert their ethnic identity. Ethnic organizations, ethnically related religious organizations, ethnically related social welfare organizations, and a variety of ethnic cultural organizations exist in major metropolitan areas of the United States. The older person can pick and choose from all of these opportunities and regain a sense of identity based on an ethnic culture.

Unfortunately, among groups defined on the basis of racial characteristics, a positive sense of in-group belonging may have to contend with a negative view of the racial group among outsiders. Although this is not true of Swedes and Italians, it is certainly an obstacle faced by African Americans of all ages. An older African American man or woman, strongly affiliated with African American culture and organizations, may come face-to-face with the problems of discrimination and hostility from Whites. The sense of belonging, achieved through new identification and participation in the African American community, may make this hostility bearable.

Immutability or Emergence

Age is an ascribed or immutable characteristic (Cell 5, Fig. 1.2) that encompasses the removal of the individual from the workforce. Ethnicity has some aspects of immutability in the racial characteristics of African Americans, Asians, and Native Americans, who are identified by society on the basis of skin pigmentation. Cantor (1988) argues:

> Race/ethnicity, like gender, is an immutable given at birth that largely determines the physical, psychosocial and personal resources with which people arrive at the threshold of old age. Being black, therefore, conditions responses to the environment and age-related changes over the later part of the life cycle. And research suggests that being black involves a whole host of related risks—the risk of poverty, chronic illness, and even death. (p. 133)

The skin color of an individual is immutable, but the cultural characteristics associated with skin pigmentation may be alterable. As already discussed, ethnic cultures change in response to a variety of conditions within their host society. Rather than being immutable, the characteristics associated with an ethnic culture can change. In turn, these emergent characteristics may affect the valuation of the culture by the dominant society (Cell 6).

Losses and Gains

The aging process is characterized by a number of losses (Cell 7), including some loss of physical functioning, the diminution of old social networks of friends and relatives through death or geographic movement, and emotional losses related to these changes. For many older persons, involvement with senior centers, clubs, new hobbies, and travel affords some compensation. Ethnic backgrounds may provide an alternative compensatory setting through a variety of ethnic organizations, as well as involvement in social issues that affect the ethnic community (Cell 8).

Involvement in the African American community can offer an entire new set of roles and statuses for the older person. The roles may be found in the African American church, mentoring of younger African Americans, civil rights activities, and many of the types of activities promoted through federal organizations such as ACTION. There are similar possibilities available for older persons from other ethnic backgrounds. Cuellar (1978) describes a situation of a low-income Latino who acquired new status as a poet after his retirement.

Adaptation

As social or physical changes take place, the older person is required to adapt (Cell 9). Adaptation means learning to cope with some physical disability and finding new activities to replace former work routines. Many ethnic cultures provide means of adaptation (Cell 10) through well-defined roles for older persons, including roles in the family and the community. The older person may be the family decision-maker. Alternatively, older people may be viewed as responsible for the passing on of important ethnic traditions.

NEGATIVE ASPECTS OF ETHNICITY

Change as Threatening

The positive elements of any model usually contain the seeds of less favorable elements. For the older person who has grown up in a strong traditional ethnic culture, the changes that they perceive within this culture may be viewed as threatening. The changes may not be seen as a means of allowing the ethnic culture to adapt to the changes in the host environment, but as a threat to the culture's very survival. The older person may make an effort to resist the changes. Resistance can take the form of demands for maintenance of traditional roles or traditional behavior patterns among family members.

An instance of this reaction was found in focus groups among Australian women who were caregivers for older parents (McCallum & Gelfand, 1990). The older parents felt that their grandchildren did not exhibit appropriate respect toward them. The grandparents also viewed the lifestyles of their Australian-born grandchildren as unsuitable. These views created conflicts within the families. In part, these can be seen as expected intergenerational conflicts; however, the conflicts may also have intensified because the grandparents viewed their adolescent grandchildren as violating cultural norms. These violations represented an undermining of the ethnic culture and a loss of ethnic values and behavior patterns. Faced with that prospect, the grandparents attempted to impose their ethnic behavioral norms, without support from their adult, more acculturated children.

An unwillingness to learn the language of the host country may also represent resistance to what the older individual regards as the loss of traditional norms. Stevens and Swicegood (1987) have noted that the willingness of an individual to become at least bilingual indicates an intent to become part of the host society. The effort to maintain the mother tongue may assist in the preservation of the ethnic culture. Unfortunately, it may harm the ability of ethnic group members to obtain adequate information about changes taking place in the host society and the impending impact of these changes on the ethnic culture.

ETHNICITY AS ROOTS

As shown in Figure 1.2, ethnicity allows the older person to identify with something not otherwise found in a homogeneous society. This motive can be seen in the efforts of individuals to put down roots.

Geographic Community and Roots

Roots can be established in a residential community. As many suburban residents will attest, however, identification with the geographic community has become more difficult in the United States, because of changes in living styles and occupational patterns. With higher education and more white collar and managerial jobs, individuals expect to move in order to advance in their careers. Facing a series of career and geographical moves, many workers may not want to put down roots, in order to avoid disappointment when job changes necessitate a move to another community. Instead, they delay any community involvement with the rationale that, after retirement, they will settle down.

There is often less geographic movement among blue collar workers. In working-class communities, job mobility is less dependent on a willingness to move. The cost of housing also limits the ability of many working-class families to move. In these communities, loyalty and commitment to the area may be greater and linked to a strong ethnic attachment. Attachment to the ethnic makeup of the community and a lack of financial means to move have been found to retard the out-migration of families when new ethnic groups begin to rent or purchase homes (Gelfand, 1973).

Occupations and Roots

As an alternative to identification with the local community, a sense of identification can be found in an occupation. This type of identification is most common among professionals. Lower-income individuals may feel that their job is merely a means of survival. For middle- and upper-income workers, however, the job often represents a career, rather than merely a salary. These workers may invest extensive emotional energy in their jobs.

Historically, a greater diversity of ethnic backgrounds has typified occupations that require advanced training. Less-skilled industrial jobs have tended to be ethnically related, because immigrants, their families, and friends could obtain these jobs soon after they arrived in the United States. Poles were strongly represented in the steel mills, Italians in construction, and other groups in a variety of unskilled labor occupations.

Family and Roots

For many individuals, the family provides the most vital roots in their lives. After World War II, some sociologists argued that the extended family was losing its importance in the United States. They believed that the nuclear family of husband, wife, and children would become the dominant family pattern. This analysis has not proven adequate. Although the nuclear family is important, there remain important relationships between extended family members, which are often apparent when an older person requires assistance. The model of the nuclear family, based on spouses and child, is also inadequate to describe families comprised of same-sex partners or families headed by single parents, particularly female headed households.

This analysis does not rule out the identification of the individual with the larger units of society, such as a city, state, or nation. In small towns and cities, identification with the political unit is not only feasible, but offers opportunities for involvement and participation. In larger communities, identification with the city or county may simply mean participation on specific topics or voting in regularly scheduled elections.

Life-Cycle Changes

Each of the most viable forms of identification undergoes changes during the life cycle. Individuals who move frequently during their younger years may plan for their retirement and discuss where to live during their later years. More well-to-do individuals may even purchase property in a community that they regard as offering a desirable place to settle and develop roots.

Retirement may lessen identification with an occupation. Former employees find that, although seemingly essential to the running of the company or office, replacing them with new employees has been possible. There may be residual identification with the firm, but little day-to-day involvement with the former work environment.

Family roots never disappear. Their intensity lessens over time, as children leave home and begin to develop their own careers and families. Contact is maintained by parents and children by visits, writing, and telephone. Day-to-day involvement of the nuclear family members in each other's lives diminishes because of reduced personal contact. Parents become less involved in their children's decision-making, unless personal crises are encountered. All of these changes may create a desire for some new attachments among older persons. Ethnic organizations or affiliations are one possible mechanism for the development of these attachments.

Ethnic Cultures and Change

The ethnic culture an 80-year-old person wants to affiliate with is likely to differ in many important ways from the culture that existed when they were a child. Public awareness of these changes may be minimal, particularly if negative attitudes toward these ethnic groups are strong. Some of these changes were necessary to enable the culture to survive in the new society; other changes were by choice.

Ethnic cultures change at different rates, according to the permeability of the culture to internal and external influences. Some changes may involve a reevaluation of the appropriate role for the older person in the church, ethnic community, or family. In Chinese communities, older persons have traditionally occupied positions of power and influence. As the existence of Chinese communities began to be threatened by urban renewal plans, such as in Boston in the 1970s, there was a movement away from the traditional older leadership. This change was necessary, because many of the older leaders could not speak English well enough to negotiate with local Boston politicians. Events of this nature can produce a permanent shift in cultural values concerning the role of the elderly.

Change is ongoing within ethnic groups. A portrayal of ethnic culture should be seen as only a snapshot of the culture at one point in time. Unfortunately, most portrayals of ethnic culture have tended to assume that the cultural landscape captured at that time represents an unchanging fixed reality. In addition to the change in the ethnic culture, there is also change in the culture of the mother country from which the ethnic culture originates. Kitano (1969) cites the puzzlement of Japanese Americans who return to Japan after living many years in the United States, only to find that the country has changed dramatically. These changes include not only massive industrialization and urbanization, but also a shift in cultural values reflected in family patterns.

Intergenerational Cultural Transmission

In order to survive, ethnic culture must be transmitted from one generation to another. One important method of transmitting ethnic values is through defining allowable and acceptable behavior for children, such as appropriate terms of respect for grandparents and obligations that the children have to the family as a whole. A second method of transmission is through setting an example, and, in behavioral terms, serving as a role model.

The Ethnic Neighborhood

Reinforcement of norms and behaviors is one of the major functions of the ethnic neighborhood. Parents may be the positive ethnic role models for children, but other residents of the community reinforce these roles. This reinforcement takes place explicitly and implicitly. Explicit reinforcement is carried out by individuals who inform children about the appropriate way to behave, or scold them when they behave in a manner inconsistent with the values of the ethnic group. Implicit and equally valuable reinforcement of ethnic norms occurs when children see the way ethnic group members relate, for example, in the maintenance of disabled older relatives at home rather than in nursing homes.

Older people have a vital role to play in the transmission of ethnic culture. They transmit the culture not only by verbal explication or through writing but also by serving as role models. These roles may include behaviors that prescribe behavior for an individual of a certain age, including attitudes about illness and death.

Implicit and explicit reinforcement of ethnic norms can be an ongoing process. One valuable example is provided by MacLean and Bonar's (1983) case study of a 93-year-old Greek widower who had been in a Montreal nursing home for 12 years, but who had had only limited contact with his children, grandchildren, and great-grandchildren since his institutionalization:

> He spends most of his time in bed, seems to feel that he is not much use to anyone, and tends to be dependent on the staff for most of his physical and social needs. This is probably mainly due to the language barrier that exists between him and the other patients. In short, Mr. C. has very little contact with anyone in the institutions.
>
> However, during the past year, Mr. C. has been befriended by a member of the auxiliary staff who is also Greek. She volunteered some extra time to listen to him and do instrumental tasks for him. During this process, she became aware of his personal circumstances. She became outraged that Mr. C. seemed to have been abandoned by his family and by the Greek community of Montreal. Her anger led her to telephone a popular Greek radio talk show where she identified the individual and his family and expressed her opinion on this kind of behavior of the Greek community toward one of its older people. This telephone call immediately mobilized Mr. C.'s family to visit him in order to make amends with him and to restore their status within the Greek community. Furthermore, the Greek community felt a sense of responsibility toward Mr. C. and several Greek volunteers now visit him on a regular basis. This has allowed Mr. C. to become re-involved with his family and his community to the extent that his social well-being is considerably improved. (MacLean & Bonar, 1983, pp. 57–58)

The Ethnic Enclave

Besides strong reinforcement of ethnic norms, there are a number of other possible and valuable functions that the ethnic community can perform. The ethnic community often functions not only as a geographic place in which a large number of individuals from a particular ethnic neighborhood live, but also as an *ethnic enclave*. As defined by Portes (1981), an ethnic enclave provides job opportunities for its residents. The ability of the enclave to provide employment for members of the ethnic group has a number of important functions. First, these jobs maintain the integration of the individual in a community where they feel comfortable. Second, the enclave shields ethnic group members from job discrimination that stems from a lack of fluency in English or from discrimination against people of minority ethnic and racial backgrounds. Third, an ethnic enclave offers opportunities for people to interact using their mother tongue and to develop relationships based on common ethnic values. A service-delivery system, attuned to the health, social, and emotional needs of members of the ethnic culture, may develop within the enclave and provide jobs for members of the ethnic group.

Institutional Completeness

If a community is large enough, it may approach what Breton (1964) has termed *institutional completeness,* a term by which he refers to a community's economic, political, and social welfare entities. These range from banks to hospitals and social services. To obtain institutional completeness, a community must meet a number of requisites, most important of which are probably population size and economic resources. Size is a requisite because a small community population cannot provide enough potential clients to make cost efficiency possible. Stores, banks, and other retail operations also have difficulty generating the profits necessary for survival.

From cursory observations, it would appear that there is institutional completeness in many ethnic communities, since a wide variety of retail establishments, banks, and social, health, and religious organizations are present. These appearances may be deceiving. The retail establishments may only be part of larger chains, and, although staffed by members of the ethnic community, nonethnics may actually own these stores. The social, health, and religious services that are present may also be only part of larger social and health organizations, and there may be little indigenous influence reflected in the local churches. In turn, attention to the specific needs of the ethnic group may be limited. As is discussed in chapter 6, these specific needs may be most important in the delivery of adequate health and social services.

Ethnicity and Heterogeneous Neighborhoods

A more problematic situation may occur if the geographically based ethnic community disappears. There are not yet indications that all ethnic communities are disappearing, but studies in the 1960s and 1970s indicated that neighborhoods comprised of White ethnics were aging, which means that the age cohort of 25- to 44-year-old individuals was underrepresented, and that older age cohorts were overrepresented. When the childbearing (25–44) age cohort is absent or underrepresented, replacement of a population is not possible. In African American, Latino, and Asian neighborhoods, this aging process is not yet taking place.

In ethnically heterogeneous communities, it is imperative for adherents of ethnic culture to develop a mechanism to communicate ethnic norms and values. A number of possible mechanisms exist for transmission of ethnic cultures. These include the establishment of ethnic journals that focus on ethnic culture. Cultural programs in schools can be instituted. Residents of heterogeneous neighborhoods can also be encouraged to attend churches that are ethnically based, even if they require travel out of the neighborhood. In Australia, ethnic clubs, such as the Hellenic Club or the Croatian Club, play a positive anchoring role in preservation of the ethnic culture. Despite these efforts, the maintenance and transmission of ethnic culture is a complex and difficult process, once the geographically based ethnic community is dispersed.

RESEARCH ON THE ETHNIC AGED

Clarification of the role of ethnicity in the lives of older people, their families, and the larger society offers a sizable research agenda. An equally important research agenda exists regarding programs and services for the ethnic aged. With such a variety of basic and applied concerns requiring investigation, why progress has been slow is difficult to understand. One simple explanation is that the needs of undifferentiated White elderly have been seen as predominant and that individuals and institutions in control of research funds reflect this attitude. This explanation is valid, but incomplete.

Leveling and Research

It would also be easy to argue that there has simply been a general lack of interest in differentiating among older people. To some extent, the age-as-a-leveler model has resulted in a general feeling that the issues facing older people are the same, with health issues being primary. Even if health issues are the most crucial for older people, clearly genetic backgrounds, environmental conditions, and access to health care result in varied health statuses among the minority and ethnic aged. Belief in a uniform aging process began to change in the late 1960s, as attention focused more on the problems of poverty in the United States. What became evident was that older people, particularly older minorities, were among the poorest of the poor.

In many research projects, minority aged are used as control variables for studies of White elderly. Studies that use African American aged, Latino aged, or even Polish aged, to highlight variations from the majority group of interest, have limited utility. What is missing from most of this earlier research is a strong interest in each of the minority populations, as well as the large number of ethnic aged from European backgrounds.

Part of the failure, or disinterest, in exploring the rich variation among Whites from varied ethnic backgrounds stems from a feeling that past differences no longer exist, and that the assimilation process has completed its work. Until recently, researchers may have been embarrassed to note ethnic differences, feeling the need to portray America as a country without any major racial or ethnic disparities. A portrayal of this kind is impossible in the 2000s, as racial and ethnic issues remain front-page headlines.

The Conduct of Research

To express an interest in racial and ethnic differences is not the same thing as carrying out adequate research that highlights differences as well as similarities. There are many difficulties, the most apparent being language issues. Research with various Latino, Asian, and European elderly confronts the researcher with the need to translate the research instruments, whether these are self-administered questionnaires or interviews. The process of translation has become fairly standardized in research methodology. The instrument is first translated into the foreign language, then translated back into English by a different person. The researcher then compares the original English version with the retranslated version, to be sure that the meaning of the items was not changed during the original translation process. The necessary revisions are then made to ensure accuracy of the translation.

This seemingly clear-cut process unfortunately contains many pitfalls. First, it assumes that there is only one agreed-upon version of any language. But, even in Spanish, word usage by Argentines, Mexicans, Cubans, and Peruvians may differ. The choice of terminology by the translator may be appropriate to one group, but not correctly understood by other Latino elderly. Even the correct choice of words for a literal translation does not signify that the meaning of the term has been understood. As every student of foreign languages quickly finds out, there are words that are untranslatable and idioms that have peculiar meanings in a language. A good example is an item on the well-known "General Well-Being" scale (Rumbaut, 1985). This item inquires about how long the respondent has been "blue." Although this term may have meaning for most Americans in a mental health context, its noncolor meaning is not connoted in other languages.

Beyond the meaning of specific terms, even a concept such as mental health or depression may not be relevant in other cultures. In some cultures, mental health problems are viewed as rooted in organic problems. No distinction is made between physical and emotional symptoms. An effort to determine comparative mental health statuses of many ethnic groups, using the same instrument, even when translated with care, may be doomed to failure.

Research and Access

A well-designed instrument, carefully crafted and attuned to the cultures being investigated, does not guarantee the success of the research. The ethnic background of the researcher may help them obtain access to the community, but this is not always true. Even if the researcher comes from the same ethnic or racial background as the prospective respondents, class differences may prevent the researcher from fully understanding what the respondent is saying. In research on stigmatized behavior such as alcohol abuse, there are also questions as to whether the research subjects are answering honestly or selecting socially desirable responses.

Older immigrants may find research questions a new experience. No matter how often the researcher assures them of confidentiality, the research may remind some immigrants of interrogations by unfriendly police in their home country. Some older persons, particularly recent immigrants, have never experienced the types of questionnaires and structured interviews so common in social science research (Gelfand, 1986). The importance of completing all questions, to ensure the viability of scales, or even how to select an answer from multiple choices, compounds the difficulty of research with these ethnic populations.

Culturally valid translations of concepts and words, and access to the community, are all important issues, but perhaps the most difficult problem for researchers is that of sampling. Research in ethnic/minority aging often uses a *convenience sample*, which Henry defines as "a group of individuals who are readily available to participate in a study" (1990, p. 18). The use of this type of sample often represents the researcher's frustration at finding no other approach except to ask any older individuals, from the ethnic population group under scrutiny, to participate.

The basic reason for this strategy lies in the lack of any adequate base for sampling. There is no master list of individuals by racial and ethnic origin available from any source. In the case of minority groups such as African Americans, Hispanics, and some Asian groups, the researcher may be able to find neighborhoods whose residents are predominantly from one ethnic population. In these cases, a random sampling, based on households, can be undertaken either by telephone or in person, as was done in the National Survey of Black Americans (NSBA).

Drawing an adequate sample of ethnic older persons from European backgrounds is even more difficult. No lists of community residents by ancestry are available, and many neighborhoods have ethnically heterogeneous populations of White residents. Self-defined "ancestry" is now available from the U.S. Census, but the wide variation in how individuals report their ancestry raises questions about the reliability of this indicator. In most cases, researchers have dismissed the possibility of sampling among Whites by ethnic background, instead opting for a design that lumps all Whites together under a rubric such as "Anglo." The increasing numbers of Americans who consider themselves to be of multiracial backgrounds adds a new layer of complexity to research focused on ethnicity.

Selecting a sample from among individuals attending specific programs and services obviously creates problems when generalizing the results. Older people who attend senior centers may be different in many ways from their counterparts of the same age. Senior center participants may differ in their general attitudes about aging, their interest and willingness to use programs and services, their attitudes toward professionals, and their basic health and mental health statuses. The program attendees may also not be representative of the poor elderly who either do not know about the programs or have no transportation to reach them.

Controlled designs, which include samples of lower- and middle-income populations from the same ethnic group of older individuals, are needed to answer important questions about ethnicity and aging. Because of their cost and logistical problems, these types of samples are rarely utilized. More adequate samples will help to resolve the issue of whether specific behaviors represent ethnic culture or some factor related to the group's socioeconomic status. Older people who live in poor, ethnically homogeneous neighborhoods may thus not be there by choice, but because costs or discrimination have made it impossible for them to obtain other housing.

Knowledge about ethnicity and aging thus remains incomplete. In the new century, a great deal more is known about the aged from African

American, Latino, and Asian backgrounds than their counterparts from European countries. Even with the improvement in the amount of research being funded and implemented, major questions remain to be explored and answered. In subsequent chapters, some of these questions are highlighted.

REFERENCES

Alba, R. (1985). The twilight of ethnicity among Americans of European ancestry: The case of Italian-Americans. In R. Alba (Ed.), *Ethnicity and race in the U.S.A.: Towards the 21st century* (pp. 134–158). Boston: Routledge and Kegan Paul.

Alba, R. (1992). Ethnicity. In E. Borgatta & M. Borgatta (Eds.), *Encyclopedia of Sociology: Volume 2* (pp. 110–112). New York: Macmillan.

American culture. (n.d.). Retrieved December 31, 2001, from *http://www.admin. uiuc.edu/NB/98.04/marriagetipL.html*

Berlin, I. (1998). *Many thousands gone: The first two centuries of slavery in North America.* Cambridge, MA: Belknap Press.

Breton, R. (1964). Institutional completeness of ethnic communities and the personal relations of immigrants. *American Journal of Sociology, 70,* 193–205.

Cantor, M. (1988). Modernization and the Black elderly. In E. Gort (Ed.), *Aging in cross-cultural perspective: Africa and the Americas.* New York: The Phelps-Stokes Fund.

Cowgill, D. (1988). Aging in cross-cultural perspective: Africa and the Americas. In E. Gort (Ed.), *Aging in cross-cultural perspective: Africa and the Americas* (pp. 110–132). New York: The Phelps-Stokes Fund.

Cuellar, J. (1978). El senior citizens club: The older Mexican-American in the voluntary association. In B. Myerhoff & A. Simic (Eds.), *Life's career—Aging* (pp. 207–230). Beverly Hills, CA: Sage.

Erdmans, M. (1995). Immigrants and ethnics: Conflict and identity in Chicago Polonia. *Sociological Quartley, 36,* 175–195.

Gelfand, D. (1973). Influx–exodus: An exploratory study of racial integration. In D. Gelfand & R. Lee (Eds.), *Ethnic conflicts and power: A cross-national perspective* (pp. 257–265). New York: John Wiley.

Gelfand, D. (1986). Assistance to the new Russian elderly. *The Gerontologist, 26,* 444–449.

Gelfand, D., & Fandetti, D. (1980). Suburban and urban white ethnics: Attitudes towards care of the aged. *The Gerontologist, 20,* 588–594.

Glazer, N. (1957). *American Judaism.* Chicago: University of Chicago Press.

Glazer, N., & Moynihan, P. (1970). *Beyond the melting pot.* Cambridge, MA: MIT Press.

Gordon, M. (1964). *Assimilation in American life.* New York: Oxford.

Guttmann, D. (1986). A perspective on Euro-American elderly. In C. Hayes, R. Kalish, & D. Guttmann (Eds.), *European-American elderly* (pp. 3–15). New York: Springer Publishing.

Henry, G. (1990). *Practical sampling.* Newbury Park, CA: Sage.

Hochschild, A. (1975). Disengagement theory: A critique and proposal. *American Sociological Review, 40,* 553–569.

Holzberg, C. (1982). Ethnicity and aging: Anthropological perspectives on more than just the minority elderly. *The Gerontologist, 22,* 249–257.

Jarvempa, R. (1985). The political economy and political ethnicity of American Indian adaptations and identities. In R. Alba (Ed.), *Ethnicity and race in the U.S.A.: Towards the 21st century* (pp. 29–44). Boston: Routledge and Kegan Paul.

Johnson, C. (1985). *Growing up and growing old in Italian-American families.* New Brunswick, NJ: Rutgers University Press.

Kendig, H. (1988). *Social change and family dependency in old age: Perceptions of Japanese women in middle age.* Research Paper Series No. XX. Tokyo: Nihon University Population Research Institute.

Kitano, H. (1969). *Japanese Americans.* Englewood Cliffs, NJ: Prentice-Hall.

Luborsky, M., & Rubinstein, R. (1987). Ethnicity and lifetimes: Selfcontexts and situational contexts of ethnic identity in late life. In D. Gelfand & C. Barresi (Eds.), *Ethnic dimensions of aging* (pp. 35–50). New York: Springer Publishing.

MacLean, M., & Bonar, R. (1983). The ethnic elderly in a dominant culture long-term care facility. *Canadian Ethnic Studies, 153,* 51–59.

Makielski, S. (1973). *Beleaguered minorities: Cultural politics in America.* San Francisco: W. H. Freeman.

McCallum, J., & Gelfand, D. (1990). *Ethnic women in the middle.* Canberra, Australia: National Centre for Epidemiology and Population Health.

Nelson, C., & Tienda, M. (1985). The structuring of Hispanic ethnicity: Historical and contemporary perspectives. In R. Alba (Ed.), *Ethnicity and race in the U.S.A.: Towards the 21st century* (pp. 49–74). Boston: Routledge and Kegan Paul.

Portes, A. (1981). Modes of structural incorporation and present theories of immigration. In M. Kritz, C. Keely, & S. Tomasi (Eds.), *Global trends in migration.* Staten Island, NY: Center for Migration Studies Press.

Pugh, T. (2001, March 24). Intermarriages rise, reflecting U.S. changes. *Philadelphia Inquirer,* 1.

Reitzes, D. (1959). Institutional structure and race relations. *Phylon, 20,* 48–66.

Rodriguez, G. (2001, February 11). Forging a new vision of America's melting pot. *New York Times,* 4:1, 4.

Rose, A. (1965). The subculture of the aging: A framework for research in social gerontology. In A. Rose & W. Peterson (Eds.), *Older people and their social worlds* (pp. 3–18). Philadelphia: F. A. Davis.

Rumbaut, R. (1985). Mental health and the refugee experience: A comparative study of Southeast Asian refugees. In T. Owan (Ed.), *Southeast Asian mental health: Treatment, prevention, services, training and research* (pp. 433–486). Rockville, MD: National Institute of Mental Health.

Schermerhorn, R. (1970). *Comparative ethnic relations: A framework for theory and research.* New York: Random House.

Schmitt, E. (2001, March 13). For 7 million people in census, one race category isn't enough. *New York Times,* A1, 14.

Stevens, G., & Swicegood, G. (1987). The linguistic context of ethnic endogamy. *American Sociological Review, 52,* 73–82.

Vasques, J. (1986). The ethnic matrix: Implications for human service providers. *Explorations in Ethnic Studies, 9*(2), 1–22.

Wirth, L. (1945). The problem of minority groups. In R. Linton (Ed.), *The science of man in the world crisis* (pp. 347–372). New York: Columbia University Press.

Chapter Two

Ethnicity, Immigration, and the Ethnic Aged

Until the 1980s, many Americans regarded immigration as a phenomenon to be studied historically, rather than as an important part of contemporary life. Even the departure of large numbers of Cubans for Florida in the 1960s appeared to be a singular event related to Fidel Castro's ascent to power. In the 1980s and 1990s, immigration became a contentious element in American public policy. The numerical impact of immigration was clearly evident in the 1990s, when 1 million immigrants a year became residents of the United States. Rates of immigration in the 1990s were double those of the highest year of immigration in the 1900s (Camarota, 2001).

Immigration has an immediate and long-term impact on aging. Depending on the age distributions among the new immigrants, large-scale immigration may immediately modify the age configuration of the country. The long-term impact of immigration stems from the characteristics of the younger individuals who usually form the majority of immigrants. These characteristics help to predict service delivery needs in later years.

At a brief glance, American immigration policies appear to be inconsistent over time, but this interpretation is not totally accurate. Particular groups have been encouraged as immigrants, but others have been discouraged, or even barred from entry into the United States. Disentangling all of the definitions and requirements of immigration, and their political and social impact, is difficult. In order to make this effort, a brief review of American immigration history, as well as current immigration policies, is important.

CURRENT IMMIGRATION PATTERNS

Based on current estimates, approximately 1.2 million legal and illegal immigrants settle in the United States each year (Camarota, 2001). Overall, the immigrant population of the United States is growing at a rate that is six and a half times faster than that of the native-born population. Immigration is now the major factor in U.S. population growth. Immigrants and their children are estimated to account for 70% of the population growth in the country during the last 10 years (Camarota, 2001). The states with the largest number of immigrants are California, Nevada, Florida, Texas, New Jersey, Illinois, Massachusetts, Arizona, Virginia, and Michigan.

Although many of them are not recent immigrants, the 2000 census counted 30 million people born outside the United States, and there are probably many more foreign-born individuals who were missed by the census. Although the numbers are very high, the percentage of foreign-born individuals living in the country is proportionately less than it was in 1900, because of the overall increase in the American population (U.S. Census Bureau, 2001). About one fourth of the foreign-born population that emigrated to the United States before 1980 is now over the age of 65. Among those that arrived between 1980 and 1989 and those that arrived in the 1990s, the percentages are 5.6 and 3.2, respectively. The median age of foreign-born individuals is now over 52, which means that, during the next 15 years, many more foreign-born individuals will join the ranks of the elderly. The largest group of foreign-born individuals who arrived in the United States during the 1980s was in the 35–44 age category. Among the foreign-born who arrived in the 1990s, the largest age group was the 25–34 age category. These individuals spent their formative years in another country (U.S. Census Bureau, 2001).

Immigrants from Europe represent 15% of the current foreign-born population. The 25.5% of the foreign-born who have emigrated from Asia and the 51% who have emigrated from Latin America overshadow this percentage. Mexicans comprise 27.6% of this latter group (U.S. Census 2002). The growth of substantial numbers of individuals from Asia, Latin America, and, to a lesser degree, Africa, has added to the diversity of the United States. In 1980, the census added a question asking people about their ancestry. Answers to this question reveal something about attitudes toward ethnic backgrounds. In the 2000 census, 20 million people stated that their ancestry was "United States or American," although their parents or grandparents may have been émigrés from other countries. As expected, 46 million people responded that they were from German ancestry, 28 million from British ancestry, 33 million from Irish ancestry, 16 million from Italian ancestry, and 10 million from French ancestry. Perhaps surprising to many Americans is the fact that 1.3 million people cited their ancestry as Arab, almost 2 million as West Indian, and 1.5 million as sub-Saharan African (U.S. Census Bureau, 2000).

In 2000, immigrants accounted for almost 13% of the total work force. Unfortunately, many of these immigrants were working in low-paid jobs. For some immigrants, this situation may result because they are undocumented workers. For many others, their lack of advanced education limits their employment possibilities. More than one third of immigrants in the work force, between 1990 and 1999, had no high school degree, and one fourth had only completed high school (Camarota, 2001). In an American economy in which well-paying factory jobs have been disappearing, limited education creates problems for immigrants and nonimmigrants seeking work.

AMERICAN IMMIGRATION HISTORY

Each group of immigrants in the United States has a distinctive history that shapes their attitudes and behaviors. Although *immigrant* is a generic term, there are three important subgroups among current immigrants to the United States: (1) individuals who have a visa to officially immigrate, (2) refugees fleeing from persecution in their native country, and (3) individuals who enter the country illegally, for a variety of reasons. During most of American history, certain countries have predominated as sources of immigrants: Germany, Great Britain, Italy, Ireland, Russia, and Austria-Hungary. Since the 1960s, this pattern has changed dramatically, with Central Americans and Asians now the most notable immigrant populations.

Early Immigration to the United States

Early English and Dutch settlers expanded the ethnic diversity of America by importing Africans as slaves as early as 1619. The slave trade, however, ended in 1801, and all states north of the Mason-Dixon line had banned slavery by 1804. As Wilson (1973) notes, a high birth rate among slaves in the United States contrasted with the low birth rate among slaves in Latin America. The higher birth rate reduced the need to import slaves. By the period immediately preceding the Civil War, the majority of slaves in the country had been born on plantations in the South. As smaller numbers of African immigrants arrived, replenishment of the various African cultures that were resident in the United States was diminished. The sale of slaves within the country also separated individuals from the same African tribes. Slaves and their children were more affected by the developing American culture. African American culture began to emerge.

The planters who first imported Africans for slavery represented a homogeneous society of predominantly British origin. Not until the period between 1820 and 1840 did the first major influx of non-British immigrants arrive at Atlantic coast ports. Despite the large number in that immigration, there was a common Anglo-Saxon background among those Irish and German immigrants. The Irish immigrants introduced a sizable Catholic population to the developing country. Anti-Catholicism quickly became a major strain in American thinking and "Irish need not apply" a common refrain in employment advertisements.

Although the industrial revolution produced economic upheavals that encouraged emigration, it was the development of the steamship that allowed massive immigration to take place. With the industrialization of the United States after the Civil War, the first group of Asians—Chinese laborers—were brought in to work on the railroads.

Mass Immigration into the United States

The years from 1880 to 1900 witnessed an increase in the number of immigrants (from approximately 450,000 to 750,000) and an increase in the diversity of the American population. For the first time, Italians, immigrants from Russia, and other groups from Southern and Eastern Europe, were represented in a tangible way in the United States.

This same pattern continued into the early 1900s. During this period, the numbers of immigrants increased even more dramatically, to over 1 million a year. Between 1900 and 1910, 8.8 million immigrants were admitted to the United States. During that decade, 1907 stands out as the highest single year of immigration.

Institution of the Quota System

Restrictions were placed on Chinese immigrants in 1882 and on Japanese immigrants by 1907. The National Origins Act of 1924 expanded the restrictive quality of American immigration policies. This act established quotas for admissions of immigrants from every country. The quotas were based on the percentage of the population from a country counted by the census of 1900. Because of the limited numbers of Eastern and Southern Europeans in the country at that time, the quota system made obtaining immigration visas difficult for individuals from countries such as Russia, Poland, Italy, and Greece.

The onset of the Depression in 1929 reduced demand for admission to the United States from Europe. In 1932, the number of immigrants dropped to below 100,000 for the first time since 1842. The closing off of massive immigration, through the quota system and the Depression, reduced the consistent flow of cultural influences from the "mother country," and increased the Americanization of the population. Following the end of World War II, there was an increase in immigration. Because of the quota system, the numbers of immigrants never reached earlier peaks, and the diversity of the immigrants remained limited.

The Preference System

The Immigration Act of 1965 repealed the quota system, which had been discredited for many years. The quota system also created major problems in the admission of refugees from Europe during World War II, the foreign brides of U.S. servicemen stationed abroad, Hungarians who fought in the 1956 uprising against the Soviet government, and Cubans who fled their country after Fidel Castro came to power.

The 1965 act completely revised the American approach to immigration. Rather than a discriminatory quota system, the act emphasizes both the reunification of families and preferences based on employment needs in the United States. At a minimum, the limits for individuals admitted under family preferences, in April 2002, was 226,000 and under employment preferences, was 140,000. However, immigrants from any one country cannot exceed 7% of the total annual allotment (*Visa Bulletin*, 2002). The allocation of the slots is based on a preference system. The preferences for family reunification are:

1st preference:	unmarried sons and daughters 21 or older of citizens
2nd preference:	**A:** spouses and children (who are under 21 and unmarried) of legal permanent residents **B:** unmarried sons and daughters (21 years of age and older) of legal permanent residents
3rd preference:	married sons and daughters of citizens

4th preference: brothers and sisters of adult citizens (*Visa Bulletin*, 2002)

Parents of U.S. citizens over the age of 21 are not subject to numerical limitations. In 1996, approximately 67,000 people over the age of 60 were admitted legally into the country. This accounted for 7% of all legal immigrants in that year.

The employment-based preferences are:

1st preference: Priority workers
2nd preference: Members of professions holding advanced degrees or persons of exceptional ability
3rd preference: Skilled workers, professionals, and other workers
4th preference: Certain special immigrants
5th preference: Employment creation (*Visa Bulletin*, 2002)

The family preferences for countries such as India, Mexico, and the Philippines had been filled long before 2002. Individuals from India, being admitted to the United States under the family preference, had filed their application for this preference before March 15,1989 (*Visa Bulletin*, 2002).

The adoption of this preference system has dramatically increased the percentage of immigrants from Asia and North and South America, but has reduced the representation of European immigrants, because they are unable to qualify under many of the preferences. The Immigration Act of 1990 altered the system by tripling (to 140,000) the number of immigrant visas allotted to managers, professionals, and others whose skills are deemed as needed in the United States. At the same time, the total immigrant quota was raised to 700,000, an increase of 40%.

There is also a diversity category under current immigration law. This category was instituted in the 1990s, as a response to complaints from individuals of ethnic backgrounds that the family preference system was unfair to many countries. Under the diversity category, preference is given to countries that are not current principal sources of immigration. The maximum number of individuals admitted under this category is 55,000. However, in 1997, Congress specified that 5,000 of these visas must be allotted to Central Americans. Allocation of the immigrant visas is on a lottery basis. In May 2000, individuals whose lottery numbers were below those indicated for each region were eligible for immigrant visas: Africa, 12,800; Asia, 7,800; Europe, 12,800; Bangladesh, 3,790; North America (Bahamas), 8; Oceania, 375; South America and the Caribbean, 940 (*Visa Bulletin*, 2002). The demand for these visas is much greater than the amount allocated. In 1997, for example, there were 7.6 million applicants for the 55,000 visas. Even with a low number, applicants must show that they have a high school degree or two years of experience working in a skilled occupation (Vaughan, 1997). Individuals from countries such as Mexico, Philippines, India, China, the Dominican Republic, Taiwan, and South Korea did not qualify for the diversity lottery, because of the high numbers of individuals from these countries already living in the United States.

Immigration and Ethnic Identity

Immigration history has enormous importance for the field of aging in the United States. The period of time during which ethnic groups arrived in significant numbers affects their proportion in the overall cohort of aged. Since Asian immigration is relatively new, many Asian Americans, regardless of age, will be first-generation immigrants. If immigrants enter the United States as adults, the influence of their ethnic culture will be stronger than if they had arrived in the country as children. Adults will have grown up in the ethnic culture and internalized cultural expectations about behavior and norms. Adjustment to the new culture is often more difficult for older immigrants than it is for younger persons. In New York City, it was clear that most of the older Russian Jewish refugees who had entered the country in the 1970s were unlikely to become proficient in English (Gelfand, 1986). In contrast, an individual who immigrates to the United States when they are young is likely to undergo a much more extensive process of acculturation, which includes not only becoming fluent in English, but also internalizing American values.

Among groups that are strongly represented in recent immigration flows, the American-born cohort will be smaller than among groups represented earlier in American immigration history. Among groups such as the Irish, the percentage of American children and grandchildren, and even great-grandchildren, is higher. Because of the historical changes in the immigration laws, age and immigration cohorts are not necessarily synonymous. Poles who are 70 years old may be the children of immigrants. Chinese of the same age are more likely to be foreign-born, because of the restrictions on Chinese immigration that existed until 1965.

Although they are certainly immigrants, individuals who enter the United States as refugees are part of a unique political category. Restrictive immigration policies have encouraged many attempts to obtain admission to the United States as refugees, rather than through the regular immigration process.

Refugee Admission Criteria

Despite the large numbers of refugees from World War II who requested refugee status, the definition used by American immigration authorities was not comparable to the international definition, until the Refugee Act was enacted in 1980. Under that legislation, refugees suffer from "a well-founded fear of persecution" if they return to their home country.

There are limits on the number of refugees that the United States will accept in any one year. This number is based on a recommendation by the President to the Congress. In 1981 (the first year that the Refugee Act was in force), the Castro government in Cuba allowed approximately 100,000 Cubans to leave the country from the port of Mariel. This group of refugees exceeded the total number of refugees targeted for the entire year by the American government. A special "parole" designation had to be utilized to allow these "Marielitos" to remain in the United States. In 2002, the numerical goal set for refugee admissions was 70,000 (*Refugee Reports*, 2001).

Beyond the issue of numbers, the ability to prove a well-founded fear of persecution is not always easy. In many cases, the decisions appear to be based on the political alliances of the United States, rather than on the individual realities of the applicants' lives. Vietnamese automatically receive refugee status, but Central Americans find that proving they are not economic migrants is difficult. Haitians, many of whom began to leave their country after the 1981 Marielito exodus, are not granted refugee status, despite the political turmoil in that island country.

Refugee and Asylee Admissions

During the 1970s, there was more than a doubling in the number of refugees, compared to the previous decade. Among European refugees, the increase was reflected in the number of individuals from the Soviet

Union, many of whom were Russian Jews. Among Asians, the increases were among Taiwanese, mainland Chinese, and Southeast Asians, particularly Vietnamese. Beginning in 1975, Vietnamese refugees, and refugees from other Southeast Asian countries, swelled the refugee totals. Cubans accounted for the largest number of individuals from Central and South America, and only small numbers of Africans were permitted to receive refugee designation.

There was an increase in the number of refugees during the 1980s. Many of the patterns of the 1970s continued, except for the substantial numbers of Iranians admitted in response to the overthrow of the Shah. The numbers of Cambodians, Laotians, and Vietnamese increased dramatically, but, except for Cubans, the numbers of Central and South Americans remained low. Among Africans during that time period, only Ethiopians were considered refugees.

The ethnic backgrounds of the refugees are substantially different from those of people entering the United States as regular immigrants. In 1999, for example, there were 85,000 people who entered the country as refugees. Of this total, 23,000 were from Bosnia and Herzegovina, 14,000 from Yugoslavia, and 17,000 from former republics of the Soviet Union. The remaining refugees were from Vietnam, Cuba, and African and Middle Eastern countries. The ethnic background of the refugees is also markedly different from the overall composition of immigrants of the early 1900s (Immigration and Naturalization Service, 2000).

Asylees are individuals who are already physically present in the United States and who then claim asylum under the same grounds as refugees. In 1999, there were 33,000 claims for asylum. The five major countries from which these applicants emigrated were China, Somalia, Haiti, Indonesia, and Mexico. Fifty-six percent of the applicants for asylum were male (Immigration and Naturalization Service, 2000).

ILLEGAL IMMIGRATION AND THE UNITED STATES

Over 420,000 individuals enter the United States annually without immigrant visas, but this number is reduced by deaths, out-migrations and legalization. The total illegal population is thus estimated to grow at a rate of 275,000 individuals each year (Center for Immigration Studies, 2000). To a large extent, these illegal immigrants are representatives of countries where the United States is loath to designate would-be immigrants as refugees. This is particularly true of Central and South American countries.

The numbers of illegal aliens currently in the United States is certainly impressive, but the out-migration data indicates that, on any given day, the figures may represent different individuals. Many of the undocumented individuals in the country on any one day may not be there the next morning. Some may be arrested by the Immigration and Naturalization Service and deported to their home country. Others may leave voluntarily. During their stay in the United States, they earned enough money to take care of their families back home for some length of time, particularly given favorable exchange rates for the U.S. dollar. There is thus a constant ebb and flow of illegal immigrants across the porous U.S. border.

Immigration Reform and Illegal Immigration

In 1986, after much debate, the Immigration Reform and Control Act (IRCA) was passed by Congress and signed by President Reagan. This legislation was an effort to control illegal immigration through both rewards and sanctions. One reward was that any individual who had been in the United States continuously, prior to January 1, 1982, was allowed to apply for amnesty and legalization. Agricultural workers were required to prove only 90 days residence between May 1985 and May 1986.

The sanctions were a new system designed to penalize employers who hire illegal immigrants. Employers are required to have new hires submit evidence documenting the workers' legal status. These documents must be kept on file for 3 years. Employers who violate this requirement are subject to an escalating series of fines and imprisonments. With this method in place, it was hoped that the incentive for men and women to come illegally to the United States to seek work would be reduced, since their job opportunities would be reduced.

The opportunity to apply for amnesty lasted from May 1987 through May 1988. During that period, over 2 million persons applied to legalize their status. Over half of the applications were received in California, and, nationally, over 70% of the applicants were Mexicans. Salvadorans and Dominicans comprised other large groups of applicants. In Maryland, the only state to undertake a study during the application period, 75 countries were represented among the applicants (Gelfand, 1989). Many of the African applicants had arrived in the United States under student visas, and stayed on illegally when their college education was completed. Haitians were also represented in substantial numbers, many working in the chicken-processing factories in the state. Nationally,

Haitians were more highly represented among the agricultural workers applying for amnesty.

Illegal Immigration Impacts

As in the case of refugees, illegal immigration brings a representation of some cultures into the United States not seen in any major proportion in the regular immigration process. Since many of these illegal immigrants stay a few months to earn money, then return to their home country, their impact on the United States is often considered minimal. This assertion is flawed.

These illegal immigrants who have crossed the border with their families enroll their children in local schools. These children may have special needs, because of poor education in their home country or a lack of any ability in English. Studies also indicate that the more often the worker crosses the border to find work, the greater the likelihood that they will remain in the United States permanently (Massey, 1986).

Questions have also been raised about the ability of the 1986 IRCA to restrain illegal immigration. Immediately after the passage of the IRCA, illegal immigration flows appeared to be reduced. This judgment was based on arrests at the border. The slowdown in persons attempting to cross the border appeared to be related to fears about increased border patrols and a lack of jobs. By 1989, research indicated that emphasis on employer sanctions in the IRCA was not having its intended effect (Cornelius, n.d.). A black market in phony documentation enabled undocumented workers to obtain jobs. In 2000, a new report indicated that the IRCA had resulted in 2.7 million people becoming legalized, but had not stemmed the impact of illegal immigration. One factor was the effort of many now-legalized aliens to have their family members join them in the United States (Center for Immigration Studies, 2000). Although further changes in immigration laws may help to clarify the situation, the vast expanse of the country's borders with Canada and Mexico means that there will always be difficulty in controlling immigration.

AGING AND IMMIGRATION

Although there have never been definitive studies, historical analyses indicate that immigrants (regardless of whether they are legal immigrants, refugees, or "illegals") are probably in some ways unrepresentative of their native population. The majority of people in all countries remain attached to their native land, despite adversities. They may move within the country as economic or political conditions change, but emigration to a completely foreign land is usually not an alternative that is considered. This reluctance to leave a homeland may persist even in the face of pending disaster. Many Jews remained in Germany despite the evident hostility of the Nazi regime against them.

Immigration and Risk Taking

The risks of facing an unknown country, foreign language, and foreign culture are often seen as greater than the risk of remaining in one's homeland. Categorizing many immigrants as "risk takers" would therefore not be unfair. This risk-taking attitude stands them in good stead during the initial period of adjustment to the new country and to the demands of growing older in a new environment.

The willingness to take risks may be true of illegal immigrants, refugees, and individuals with immigrant visas. Risk-taking attitudes may be less apparent among individuals who have had to leave their homeland at an advanced age. Forced to leave because their children are departing, or brought to the new country to provide child care for the family, the older person may not view the future optimistically. As Moon and Pearl comment about older Korean immigrants:

> After spending more than a half a century fulfilling their obligation to the Confucian system of their native land, and to the elderly who preceded them, they had every reasonable expectation that their hard work and devotion would be rewarded in turn by the deference, respect, and devotion of their own children, who were products of that same system. But when they followed their children to America, they found a life very different than the one they had anticipated. They found a culture in which the elderly are not looked up to for their wisdom and dismissed as being behind the times and out of touch, in which self-actualization is held up as the ultimate goal of healthy psychological development and loyalty to self supersedes loyalty to family. A culture in which children are reared to be emotionally independent of their parents and, as they reach their own adulthood, to relate to their parents as peers rather than as authority figures; a culture to which their children, inevitably, were rapidly adapting. They found themselves burdened with feelings of alienation, the feelings of strangers in a strange land. (1991, p. 122)

Language, transportation, and cultural problems face every immigrant to a new country. For the younger immigrant, escape from persecution and the possibility of economic opportunities may be seen as both a relief and a challenge. For the older immigrant, the losses involved in emigration from their homeland may outweigh any perceived advantages of the move to the new country. The greater the discrepancy between the living style and culture of the new and old countries, the greater the loss the older individual may perceive. For example, older Hmong immigrants evidence signs of depression (Hayes, 1988). Latinos who have immigrated to the United States at an older age also report more disability and lower life satisfaction than younger persons (Angel & Angel, 1992), a finding partially explainable by the loss of social contacts during the immigration process.

Immigration may thus have a varied impact on individuals, based both on the reasons they left their country and on their age cohort. Immigrants who have elected to come to the United States may view it as a long-term change in which they are afforded opportunities that compensate for the changes in culture and lifestyles. The refugee may view immigration as a safe haven until a return to their own country. Illegal immigrants may fall into either of these two groups, depending on whether they fled civil strife or poverty.

Immigrants who are undocumented often leave their country because of political turmoil that makes it impossible for them to work or even to survive. Other undocumented immigrants attempt to enter the United States in order to earn enough money to support their families. A third group leaves their home country because they find their religious, sexual, or political self-expression thwarted under the existing political system.

Immigration and Acculturation

The reasons for emigration may affect the attitudes the individual adopts toward their new country, their mental health, and the extent to which they attempt to acculturate to their new environment. Torres-Gil (1992) describes *acculturation* as "functioning as a member of U.S. society, speaking English, participating in the political process, and integrating oneself into social and civil life. It differs from assimilation, which implies surrendering one's ethnic identity and pride" (p. 171). As Giachello (2001) notes, acculturation may be a two-step process for most immigrants. The first step includes alterations of food habits and clothing and learning of the new language. The second involves adoption of new cultural values and beliefs.

Immigrants who leave the old country by choice may work intensely to become involved with their new homeland. They may even overtly reject their old country and any association with elements of the culture.

Immigrants who are uprooted, and who flee their homes because of political and social turmoil, may never abandon the hope of returning home. This hope, no matter how unrealistic, may retard their interest in any extensive integration into a new society.

Individuals who arrive in a new country in their later years may not discern any advantage to exerting an effort to becoming involved in the new country. Basic acculturation strategies that allow them to survive in the new environment may form the boundaries of their involvement.

Extensive involvement in a new host society requires a significant commitment for individuals from cultures whose values are distant from those of Americans. As Brower (1980) notes, "To a Vietnamese family, becoming 'like an American' may mean loudness, disobedience, disrespect, and lack of concern for the elderly" (p. 651). Vietnamese refugees who perceive themselves as being in the United States for only a temporary period may not want to make accommodation to these values. They may even attempt to erect barriers that prevent these new cultural norms from invading traditional values and may reject any notion of acculturation.

Brower's comment indicates that acculturation can have both positive and negative impacts. Tran, Fitzpatrick, Berg, and Wright (1996) found more self-reported health problems among less-acculturated older Latinos. Research with Mexican students in the United States found that students who were "Mexican-oriented" reported themselves in better health and more pleased with their physical appearance than students who were more "Anglo-oriented" (Montgomery, 1992).

The elements that need to be included in any concept of acculturation have been a matter of contention. In many cases, the ability to speak, read, and write English has been defined as the primary element. Carter-Pokras and Zambrana (2001) have criticized acculturation scales as focusing too heavily on language use and place of birth. Recent acculturation research has also focused on media preferences, involvement in the ethnic culture, and ethnic backgrounds of the relationships the individual has with other people. One study, based on national data, found complex interrelationships between language acculturation, financial strain, education, and measures of psychological distress (Krause & Goldenhar, 1992). Three Latino groups were included in this research: immigrant Mexican and Cuban Americans and Puerto Ricans born in Puerto Rico.

IMMIGRATION AND DIVERSITY

As already noted, the most visible impact of current immigration flows is the increasing diversity of the population in both the United States and Canada. The estimate is that, during the next 50 years, immigration, combined with natural increases resulting from births among current residents, will fuel the expansion of the American population from 270 million to more than 400 million (Center for Immigration Studies, n.d.).

There are differences in the geographic concentrations of ethnic populations, but, as immigrants begin to move to seek better job opportunities, the ethnic diversity of most states has increased. This was already evident in the 1980s. In the small state of Rhode Island, the Asian population increased by 245% during that decade, bringing this population to over 18,000 people (Butterfield, 1991). During the 1990s, the Asian population in Michigan grew by 71% and represented almost 2% of the state's population in 2000 (Warikoo, 2001).

A young age is also associated with refugees who often endure extreme hardships. Vietnamese refugees fleeing by boat faced the possibility of attack by pirates. Among individuals with immigrant visas, there is a higher percentage of older people. These age differences are evident in a study of Chicago's ethnic populations (Gemperle & Petersen, 1989). Indo-Chinese, Filipinos, and Chinese in the survey had a median age in the 50s when they arrived in the United States, and Koreans had a median age of 63. In contrast, Mexicans and Puerto Ricans had a median age of 31 when they immigrated to the United States, which is not surprising, since many migrants enter the country in order to find work. Older individuals attempting to migrate as refugees may not want to endure the hardship associated with emigration.

THE AGING IMMIGRANT

Many in the current large population of refugees and illegal immigrants will become aged at the same time that the large so-called "baby boomers" become aged. The baby boomers will enter this period of their lives with far superior resources and functional status. A projection of the needs of refugees and illegal aliens indicates a potential crisis for providers in 30 years, or even less.

The crisis will be most acute among individuals who have remained in the country without achieving legalization of their status. Immigrants who have become citizens are eligible for the benefits of significant programs. These immigrants will have a base of benefits when they are older, including Medicare for their health needs. Immigrants who leave their country as older individuals often do so under a preference uniting families. In Australia, this family reunion preference also requires that the families provide a guarantee of support for the person, and promise to repay the government for any benefits the older person receives before they are eligible for a government pension. In the United States, there is no comparable requirement, but, if immigrants are not able to find jobs or pay for their own health insurance, family members have to provide additional support.

Cash and medical assistance programs for refugees have been reduced dramatically since the 1980s, with much of the burden for funding these programs placed on individual states. If cash assistance and medical assistance can help withstand the initial financial problems of resettlement, the psychological issues of leaving a homeland do not disappear so easily.

The same issues of financial problems and loss of homeland face illegal aliens. For illegal immigrants growing older in the United States, some problems may be intensified because of their illegal status. Among the most crucial problems for providers are health and mental health problems.

Immigrants and Health

Delineating the impact of immigration on health is made difficult because of the number of variables that have an impact on an individual's health in a new country. These include the health status of the individual before they arrive in the United States, their knowledge of the American health care system, their attitudes toward formal health care, and their eligibility for a variety of health services. As Wong (2001) emphasizes, the stresses many immigrants face include limited education, language problems, the disruption of the family caused by not all members emigrating, and a lack of a variety of economic and emotional resources to cope with difficult changes. However, even if the immigrant arrives in the country in good health, their health status may begin to deteriorate. The deterioration may be produced by the factors Wong (2001) cites. Additionally, acculturation to an American lifestyle, with negative changes in diet and increased rates of smoking and drinking, may worsen or create new health problems for immigrants. The result is that Latino newcomers tend to live longer, have less heart disease, and exhibit lower rates of breast cancer among women (Falcon, Aguirre-Molina, & Molina, 2001). Research with Asian Indian immigrants in Atlanta, between the ages of 50 and 78, found that poorer health status was associated with the following factors: not having a relative nearby, a perception that social support was not available, older age, being female, a high body mass index, and longer length of time living in the United States (Diwan & Jonnalagadda, 2001).

The situation may be different among immigrants who arrived in the United States at an older age. These older immigrants may not have had access to adequate health care in their homeland. Even if good health care was available, immigrants from lower socioeconomic backgrounds may have been unable to afford regular health care. Civil strife may also have made trips to obtain health care too dangerous.

During the early 1900s, American inspectors at Ellis Island often used poor health as an excuse to keep individuals from "undesirable" countries from entering the country. A large immigrant population that crosses borders surreptitiously is not subject to any health checks. Although fears of communicable diseases among this population have not materialized, concern about the health status of illegal immigrants should not abate. The problems of illegal immigrants are not only the health conditions which they bring with them, but also the continued unavailability of adequate care for them in the United States, because the illegal immigrant who has no health insurance to pay for physicians and hospitals often cannot afford to pay on an out-of-pocket basis.

In some cases, undocumented workers are employed in jobs in which health insurance is not offered as a benefit, or in part-time jobs, which provide no benefits. There are also cases in which health insurance is available to the employee, but the cost is seen as prohibitive, not only on an absolute basis, but also on how individuals value health insurance. Among some illegal immigrants, health insurance that costs $200 a month is a less important expenditure than using this money to support relatives who remain in Mexico or El Salvador.

Fears of applying for public programs, which might require documentation of their immigration status, inhibit their utilization of any social welfare programs. Eligibility for these programs was also restricted in 1996 to U.S. citizens, making it impossible even for individuals who had obtained permanent resident status to obtain a variety of services.

One major public facility that provides major service to illegal immigrants is the emergency room of hospitals. Faced with an increasing number of indigent patients, public hospitals have begun to restrict the hours that the emergency room is open, or even close to their emergency rooms entirely. A number of nonprofit hospitals around the country have closed their doors or have been sold to private, profit-making firms, who may not find it profitable to keep their emergency rooms in operation. In some cases, hospitals have been redesigned to serve a long-term geriatric population, or to provide other more lucrative types of services.

Clinics operated by sectarian agencies (particularly the Catholic Church), and volunteer clinics, attempt to fill the gap in health services for undocumented immigrants and their families. Despite these efforts, the health care received by illegal immigrants remains inadequate. The health care practices of a 30-year-old man or woman, and the health care services they receive at this age, play a large part in determining their health status when they reach their sixties. Based on the socioeconomic conditions of current illegal immigrants, there is reason to expect that, as they age, their functional impairments and underlying health status will be worse than current cohorts of aged.

A higher-than-normal incidence of strokes and heart disease may occur among aging illegal aliens, because of poor diets, a lack of adequate exercise, and poor working and living conditions. In addition, many physical problems will be left untreated, and some of these acute problems among younger individuals will become chronic conditions among the aged.

The costs of this poor health care will not only be borne by the older person, but by dollars American taxpayers contribute to public health facilities. The irony will be that the ineligibility of illegal immigrants for public programs will have helped to produce the high prevalence of serious chronic conditions and impairments among this population at a later date. Maintaining this ineligibility for older illegals will not reduce the severity of their health problems. Instead, the controversy will rage about who is responsible for their home care, hospital bills, adult day care costs, and nursing home stays. In 2002, hospitals were already providing an estimated $2 billion of uncompensated care for illegal residents of all ages (Canedy, 2002).

Immigrants also often do not always seek help for mental health problems. Russian immigrants to Israel preferred to use medical doctors and medical centers as mental health providers, rather than other more specifically trained professionals (Brodsky, 1988). This inclination may represent unfamiliarity with mental health services. For Vietnamese refugees, there is not only unfamiliarity with mental health services, but also with Western concepts of mental health. In addition, cultural explanations of mental health problems often do not coincide with Western interpretations.

Mental health problems can occur among all immigrants, regardless of their legal status. Illegal immigrants, attempting to access services designed to mitigate mental health problems of immigrants, face the same barriers they encounter when seeking care for physical health problems. Untreated depression among younger adults may make it impossible for them to adapt to the demands of American society as they age. Among older people, dependency, isolation, and depression create problems for the entire family.

Immigrants are an important component of the current and future ethnic aged population. As is already evident, immigrants differ in a variety of cultural and socioeconomic dimensions. Although it is possible to examine the status of the individual immigrant, a more profitable approach is to place current immigrant populations within the context of the ethnic composition of the United States. Chapter 3 provides an overview of important ethnic groups in the country, with an emphasis on the role and status of the aged within these groups.

REFERENCES

Angel, J., & Angel, R. (1992). Age at migration, social connections and well-being among elderly Hispanics. *Journal of Aging and Health, 4,* 480–499.

Brodsky, B. (1988). Mental health attitudes and practices of Soviet Jewish immigrants. *Health and Social Work, 13,* 130–136.

Brower, I. (1980). Counseling Vietnamese. *Personnel and Guidance Journal, 58,* 648–653.

Butterfield, F. (1991, Feb. 24). Asians spread across a land, and help change it. *New York Times,* A22.

Camarota, S. (2001). Immigration in the United States—2000. Washington, DC: Center for Immigration Studies. Retrieved April 15, 2002, from *http://www.cis.org/articles/2001/back101.html*

Canedy, D. (2002, August 25). Hospitals feeling strain from illegal immigrants. *New York Times,* A12.

Carter-Pokras, M., & Zambrana, R. (2001). Latino health status. In M. Aguirre-Molina, C. Molina, & R. Zambrana (Eds.), *Health issues in the Latino community* (pp. 23–54). San Francisco: Jossey-Bass.

Center for Immigration Studies. (n.d.). *Topics.* Retrieved May 17, 2001 from *http://www.cis.org/topics/current numbers.html*

Center for Immigration Studies. (2000). *New INS report: 1986 amnesty increased illegal immigration.* Retrieved May 18, 2001, from *http://www.cis.org/ins1986amnesty.html*

Cornelius, W. (n.d.). Labor migration to the United States: Development, outcomes and alternatives in Mexican sending communities. In *Unauthorized migration: Addressing the root causes, Research addendum: Vol. 1.* Washington, DC: Commission for the Study of International Migration and Cooperative Economic Development.

Diwan, S., & Jonnalagadda, S. (2001, November). Social integration and health of Asian Indian immigrants in the U.S. Paper presented at the annual meeting of the Gerontological Society of American, Chicago.

Falcon, A., Aguirre-Molina, M., & Molina, C. (2001). Latino health policy: Beyond demographic determinism. In M. Aguirre-Molina, C. Molina, & R. Zambrana (Eds.), *Health issues in the Latino community* (pp. 3–22). San Francisco: Jossey-Bass.

Gelfand, D. (1986). Assistance to the new Russian elderly. *The Gerontologist, 26,* 444–449.

Gelfand, D. (1989, Spring). Serving the newly legalized. *Public Welfare,* 25–32.

Gemperle, R., & Petersen, B. (1989). *Service utilization by Chicago's ethnic elderly.* Chicago: Department on Aging and Disability Planning Division: Research and Statistical Analysis Unit.

Giachello, A. (2001). The reproductive years: The health of Latinas. In M. Aguirre-Molina, C. Molina, & R. Zambrana (Eds.), *Health issues in the Latino community* (pp. 107–156). San Francisco: Jossey-Bass.

Hayes, C. (1988). Two worlds in conflict: The elderly Hmong in the United States. In D. Gelfand & C. Barresi (Eds.), *Ethnic dimensions of aging* (pp. 79–95). New York: Springer Publishing.

Immigration and Naturalization Service. (2000). *Refugees, Asylees, Fiscal year 1999.* Retrieved March 25, 2002, from *www.ins.usdoj.gov/graphics/aboutins/statistics/99*

Krause, N., & Goldenhar, L. (1992). Acculturation and psychological distress in three groups of elderly Hispanics. *Journals of Gerontology: Social Sciences, 47,* S279–288.

Massey, D. (1986). The settlement process among Mexican migrants to the United States. *American Sociological Review, 51,* 670–684.

Montgomery, G. (1992). Acculturation, stressors and somatization patterns among students from the extreme South Texas. *Hispanic Journal of Behavioral Sciences, 14,* 434–454.

Moon, J., & Pearl, J. (1991). Alienation of elderly Korean American immigrants as related to place of residence, gender, age, years of education, time in the U.S., living with or without children, and living with or without a spouse. *International Journal of Aging and Human Development, 32,* 115–124.

Refugee Reports. (2001). 2001 statistical issue. *22*(12), 3.

Torres-Gil, F. (1992). *The new aging: Politicians and change in America.* New York: Auburn House.

Tran, T., Fitzpatrick, J., Berg, W., & Wright, R., Jr. (1996). Acculturation, health, stress and psychological distress among elderly Hispanics. *Journal of Cross-Cultural Gerontology, 11,* 149–165.

U.S. Census Bureau. (2000). *Profile of selected Social Characteristics: 2000.* Washington, DC: Author.

U.S. Census Bureau. (2001). *Profile of the foreign-born population in the United States: 2000,* Retrieved March 21, 2002, from *http://www.census.gov/prod/2002pubs/p23-206.pdf*

U.S. Census Bureau. (2002). *March 2000, Current Population Survey.* Washington, DC: Author.

Vaughan, J. (1997, Spring). Visa lottery still an inviting option. *Immigration Review, 28,* 10–13.

Visa Bulletin. (2002). *8*(43). Retrieved March 25, 2002, from *http://travel.state.gov/visa_bulletin.html*

Warikoo, N. (2001, March 19). Asian population leaps 71%. *Detroit Free Press,* 3B.

Wilson, W. (1973). *Power and privilege.* New York: Macmillan.

Wong, M. (2001). The Chinese elderly: Values and issues in receiving adequate care. In L. Olson (Ed.), *Age through ethnic lenses: Caring for elderly in a multicultural society* (pp. 17–32). Lanham, MD: Rowman and Littlefield.

Chapter Three

Ethnic Aged in the United States

The current situation of all ethnic groups has its origins in the history of these groups. What is common to most ethnic groups within the United States is a need to overcome poverty and discrimination. African Americans have had to overcome the legacy of slavery. Native Americans have had to confront genocidal attitudes. For both groups, progress means a continued confrontation with unclear, changing, and often damaging American policies.

Representing the largest group of current immigrants into the country, Latinos currently bear the brunt of anti-immigration feeling. These feelings have their roots not only in negative attitudes and stereotypes about other cultures, but also in fears of jobs being taken away by immigrants willing to work for low wages. Asians have faced discrimination since they began arriving in the United States. This discrimination reached its height during World War II, when Japanese Americans were placed in internment camps. The attacks on the World Trade Center in September 2001, and tensions in the Middle East, increased negative attitudes and discrimination toward Arab Americans in many locations.

American ethnic groups have generally benefited from major improvements in living standards during the twentieth century. Unfortunately, these improvements have not been consistent along all dimensions and not equally distributed across all groups. A review of the economic and health status of older persons within major ethnic groups reveals the uneven quality of the improvements in standards of living.

Economic Status

The economic status of a group or an individual can be measured in a number of ways. First, of course, is the actual amount of individual income. Income statistics are often confusing. At times, they are reported in terms of individual income, and at other times as the total annual income of a household. Second, a group's average or median income can be compared to the poverty index developed by the federal government. This figure supposedly represents the cost of a market basket of food, multiplied by three. The income of any group, such as Blacks, can also be compared to that of Whites. This ratio can be charted historically to ascertain whether it has improved or worsened. Besides the actual amount of income, the sources of income need to be explored. Sources of income provide information about the history of an age cohort, as well as the ability to confront economic crises.

Health Status

Health status among older people must be measured along two important dimensions. One dimension is the objective health status of the individual, including a person's ability to carry out basic daily functions; second is the individual's perception of their health status. This second dimension stems from the fact that good or poor health has different meanings for different people. What it means to be in good health to a younger person may not be the same for an older person who has become accustomed to a variety of annoying, but not life-threatening, chronic ailments, such as arthritis. Witnessing similar problems among friends and relatives of the same age, the older person may use these individuals' health conditions as a reference point for their own physical problems.

Evaluation of health status may also be related to a specific ethnic or racial group, and based on the group's history and living conditions. African Americans or Native Americans who have low incomes and poor living conditions may view objective health problems in a more positive light than their middle-class counterparts, who have higher expectations about their health. Without delving into every possible illness, it is important to examine whether specific ethnic elderly cohorts have a higher prevalence of the major causes of mortality, such as heart disease, cancer, and stroke.

This chapter's review of the current conditions facing American ethnic groups and their older members focuses on groups that are classified by the federal government as minorities: African Americans, Latinos, Native Americans, and Asians. Unfortunately, complete comparability in the discussion is not possible, because data collection is inconsistent. Data on African Americans and Latinos are relatively available, particularly in recent years. National data on Asians are spotty, and data on Native Americans have many missing elements. If these groups present problems for this chapter, the situation for ethnic groups with European backgrounds is much worse, since no statistics are collected by federal or state agencies specifically on these groups.

AFRICAN AMERICAN AGED

"Black Americans," "African Americans," "Blacks," "Colored," and "Negroes" are some of the names that have been used to designate dark-skinned Americans. Some of these names reflect negative stereotypes and prejudice on the part of Whites. Some are based on skin color. Until the 1960s, the more respectable term was *Negro*, which supposedly reflected physical distinctions between Negroes, Caucasians, and Asians. As the Black Power movement took hold in the 1960s, the term *Black* came into common usage. This term also reflected skin color, but it was meant to be a positive statement about the pride that African Americans should feel in their history. During the 1980s, the term *African American* became important in the Black community. The adoption of this terminology has been encouraged as a reflection of the cultural distinctiveness of Blacks in the United States, and, according to its proponents, this cultural distinctiveness equals the cultural distinctiveness of Japanese Americans or Italian Americans.

African American History in the United States

African Americans in the United States have traditionally been a population whose base was in the South. This geographic identity stems from the primarily Southern location of plantation owners who used slaves. After the Civil War, there was no immediate rush of "freedmen" to move north, because of their belief that life was going to improve dramatically in the South. The efforts of the Freedmen's Bureau, the Black community itself, and other programs, indicated a commitment to major changes in the South's economic and social structure (Foner, 1988). As the hopes for Reconstruction faded, the situation facing ex-slaves grew worse. Sharecropping and Jim Crow became common features of the South. As Foner remarks, however, "The institutions created or consolidated after the Civil War—the black family, school and church—provided the base from which the modern civil rights revolution sprang" (1988, p. 612).

These institutions were not only crucial in the development of the civil rights movement that began in the 1950s, but they are also important elements in the lives of the current cohort of Black elderly. Many of these men and women are children of families who moved north to take advantages of opportunities for better jobs. These jobs were plentiful because World War I had temporarily ended the influx of Europeans into the United States. In New York City, the number of African Americans in manufacturing, mechanical, trade, and transportation doubled between 1910 and 1920. Black women, who formerly were relegated to work as domestics, found job opportunities in manufacturing (Scheiner, 1974). Despite the opening of these jobs to a greater number of African Americans, Black men and women still found themselves relegated to lower echelons of the work force and were kept out of the developing union movement.

Part of the resistance of union members was based on unfair stereotypes of African Americans as "scabs," that is, individuals who were used to break strikes. This stereotype developed during the period when manufacturers recruited African Americans from the South to move north and work in the steel mills and in the automobile plants of Detroit, particularly when the plants were being threatened by strikes. The role that these early Black industrial workers played in strikebreaking resulted in them being regarded as unsuitable union members. Although industrial unions opened their membership in later years to African Americans, the craft unions (e.g., plumbers, carpenters) used numerous means to maintain their exclusionary policies.

Backgrounds of Black Elderly

Because of job insecurity, lower income jobs, and discrimination, few of the current cohort of Black elderly enter their later years with adequate income, good health status, or higher levels of education.

In 2000, Black men and women over the age of 65 comprised just under 8% of the total Black population (U.S. Census Bureau, 2001b). Another 6.5% of the Black population is between the ages of 55 and 64. As is true in all older age groups, there are more older Black women than men. Among Black women, 8.8% are over age 65, and an additional 7.1% of Black women are between the ages of 55 and 64. Black men over the age of 65 comprise 6.6% of Black men and 5.9% of Black men are between 55 and 64 (U.S. Census Bureau, 2001b). Individuals pessimistic about the toll that alcohol abuse, drug abuse, and homicide are taking among younger Black men would predict an even greater disparity in these figures in future years. If this toll is severe, the growth rate among the Black elderly, particularly men, may be slower than now estimated. By the year 2015, the number of Black elderly is projected to reach over 4 million and, 25 years later (2040), over 8 million. Although the White older population will also be growing dramatically during this period, the growth rate for Black elderly is projected to be 241%, a figure double that of White elderly.

It is hoped that this rapidly growing population will be better situated in terms of their economic and health status than the current cohort of Black elderly. In contrast to the 7.8% of non-Hispanic White elderly who were living below the poverty level in 2001, almost one fourth of Black elderly are living below the federal poverty level (Pear, 2002). The federal poverty level ($8,860 in 2002), however, does not reflect the income necessary to maintain an adequate lifestyle in contemporary America.

The percentage of African Americans, as well as Whites, living in poverty increases with age. Among Whites, the proportions rise from 7.6%, for persons 65 to 74 years old, to 10.4% for those 75 and over. Among African Americans, the figures rise from 22.4% to over 26%. The poverty rate among African Americans over the age of 75 remains three times higher than that of their White age peers. Low or nonexistent earnings and a lack of pensions contribute to the higher poverty rates among both White and African American women.

Life Expectancy

In 1999, life expectancy for a child born in that year in the United States was 76.7 years. There were, however, still differences in the life expectancy of men and women: The life expectancy at birth for women was 79.4 years and for men was 73.9 years. Although they have lessened over the years, there are still differentials in the life expectancies of Blacks and White men and women. For White women born in 1999, life expectancy was 79.9 years, but it was 74.7 years for Black women. A White male born in 1999 could be expected to live 74.6 years, but a Black male, only 67.8 years. Despite the large gap in life expectancy between White and Black men, it is a positive change that, between

1980 and 1999, the biggest increase in life expectancy has been among Black men (Anderson & DeTurk, 2002).

Life expectancy continued to rise in 2000: A child born in that year had a life expectancy of 76.9 years. Most importantly, the gap in life expectancy between men and women and African Americans and Whites continued to narrow. In 2000, a woman's life expectancy was 5.4 years greater than a man's, and Whites had a 5.3-year advantage in life expectancy over African Americans (Associated Press, 2002).

Most men and women can now expect to live well beyond their 65th birthday. In 1999, individuals who reached the age of 65 could expect an average life expectancy of 17.7 years. White men and women could expect an average of life expectancy of 16.1 and 19.2 years, respectively. Black men and women had shorter average life expectancies (14.3 and 17.3 years). Both White and Black men and women who reach the age of 85 could expect to live an average of 5–7 years. The continued growth of the population over the age of 85 strengthens the concerns about the ability of the American social welfare system to meet the needs of this group.

Among African Americans, however, there are a number of other points that need to be highlighted concerning these life expectancy figures. There is a five-year differential life expectancy at birth between Black and White women and a seven-year differential among men. If "old age" or "elderly" has some relationship to total life span, African Americans have argued that older African Americans (and, as is shown below, older Latinos and Native Americans) deserve these designations at an earlier time. The importance of this designation is not merely rhetorical, but affects the eligibility of these ethnic elderly for federal programs and benefits.

At approximately age 72–75, a "crossover" effect in life expectancies has been found to occur between African Americans and Whites. As a result of this crossover, life expectancies of older Blacks become better than those of Whites in their 70s. One possible cause of this crossover effect is the difference in the life histories of older Blacks and Whites. Faced with racial discrimination, poorer jobs, inadequate health care, and poor residential environments, only those Black men and women who could avoid or overcome exposure to severe conditions survive into their later years. These men and women are better suited to survive the adversities facing them in later years than Whites of the same age, who have not had the same problems at earlier points in their life.

It is unclear, at present, whether the above explanation, based on mortality selection, is sufficient (Manton, 1982). Another possible explanation is the different rates of aging for Blacks and Whites. Based on this approach, there should be distinct susceptibility among Whites and Blacks to specific illnesses and causes of death.

Health Status of Black Elderly

The major causes of death among Blacks and Whites show a few differences. The top five causes of death among both groups are heart disease, cancer, stroke, chronic obstructive pulmonary disease, pneumonia and influenza, but the remainder of the top 10 causes of death vary. Most significant is that Alzheimer's disease is the ninth-leading cause of death among Whites, but is not among the "top 10" for Blacks (Administration on Aging, n.d.).

Among the major health problems facing older people, a number are more common among Blacks than Whites, including arthritis, hypertension, and diabetes. The incidence of all types of cancer, except breast cancer among females, is higher among African Americans than all other ethnic/racial groups (Jones, Hernandez-Valero, Esparza, & Wilson, 2001). Survival rates for African American cancer and hypertension patients are also lower.

Cancer mortality rates among African Americans are 20–40% higher than among Whites. Black women with hypertension are twice as likely to die from this disease than their White counterparts (Jackson & Sellers, 2001).

Although cancer is the second-leading cause of death in the United States, the most prevalent type of cancer differs by group. The prevalence rate of the four major cancer sites (lung, breast, colon, and prostate) is higher among Blacks than Whites, except for female breast cancer. The only forms of cancer in which Blacks have a higher survival rate than Whites are cancers of the nervous system and brain (myelocytic leukemia and non-Hodgkin's lymphoma) among women (Jones et al., 2001). African Americans also die more often from cancers that appear to be related to occupational hazards and poor living conditions (National Caucus and Center on Black Aged, 1989). Some of these occupational hazards are related to the movement of older African Americans from the South to work in factories where they were assigned the most dangerous jobs.

Two of the most common forms of death among Blacks do not show up in the top 10 list for Whites. These include HIV (the seventh leading cause of death among Blacks) and homicide (the eighth leading cause of death among Blacks) (Anderson, 2001). Given all of this negative data, not surprisingly, 40% of African American elderly classify themselves as in "fair" or "poor health," compared to 26% of White elderly (Ferris, 2000). The data on HIV and homicide are particularly important, because they indicate problems that will affect many younger Black men and women before they reach their later years. Because HIV patients are now living longer, it is also possible that many of these individuals will reach old age in fragile health.

Some of the deaths attributed to cancer could be prevented by changes in the occupational conditions under which people work, or in living conditions or diet. A substantial proportion of these deaths could also be prevented by early diagnosis and treatment. This is particularly true of a number of forms of cancer for which treatment and prognosis for long-term survival has substantially improved in recent years. The problems of health care delivery to the ethnic aged is examined in more detail in chapter 7.

Functional Status of Black Elderly

For many older persons, the major problems in life are conditions that are not life-threatening, but that impair their functioning. Examining the needs of older people for assistance, the census reported that, during the 1990s, 40% of older African Americans had severe functional limitations, compared to 27% of Whites (Dilworth-Anderson, Williams, & Williams, 2001). Among older Blacks, the task requiring the most assistance is housework. Among Whites, the greatest needs are for assistance with housework and getting around outside the home.

African Americans evidence greater need than Whites on every one of the indicators. The greatest differentials are in housework, personal care (such as dressing and eating), and preparing meals. Almost twice as many Black elderly as White elderly express a need for assistance in preparing meals.

Economics and Life Satisfaction

Economic data on African Americans presents a very mixed picture. The poverty rate for African Americans has dropped from a high of 33% in 1990–1991 to 22% in 2001 (Pear, 2002). There are, however, a number of additional factors that need to be considered in evaluating the status of the Black elderly. The first is that the data on Black poverty combines different age cohorts, thereby concealing significant cohort differences. With each younger cohort, there are greater levels of educational attainment and income. More than twice as many older Blacks than Whites are currently living in poverty (Table 3.1). Hopefully, the 22% of older Black men and women currently living in poverty (Table 3.1) will decline during the next decades.

Income levels and life satisfaction are not perfectly related. In many cases, older African Americans express satisfaction with their retirement years. As Johnson, Gibson, and Luckey (1990) note, this finding contradicts those who argue that the most satisfied older persons are those who remain in the work force. This reaction may stem from the low-paying jobs that Black men and women hold and their relief at not having to do these jobs any longer. A second explanation is that, with retirement, job security issues disappear and the older individual is guaranteed a Social Security check, regardless of how low this amount may be.

LATINO AGED

As is true with White elderly, Native American elderly, and even Black elderly, the term *Hispanic* is representative of a large number of groups, because it uses a common language denominator as a surrogate for a common culture. There is now strong sentiment among many Spanish-speaking populations in the United States that *Latinos* is a better term, because it reflects a cultural background, rather than a language commonality.

Distribution of the Latino Population

In 2000, Latinos accounted for 12.5% of the U.S. population. This Census Bureau figure, however, probably underestimates the total, since many undocumented Latinos were not counted in the enumeration. Latino groups are not represented equally in the United States (U.S. Census Bureau, 2001b). Among Latinos, 66% are from Mexico. The representation of older people among Latinos is substantially less than it is among Whites. Fourteen percent of Whites are over the age of 65, but only 5.3% of Latinos are in this age category. Among Cubans, however, 21% are over 65. To a large extent, these differences represent variations in the immigration patterns of these two groups: Mexicans continue to emigrate to the United States, but the major Cuban immigrations occurred in the 1960s and 1980s.

TABLE 3.1 Poverty Among Older Whites, Blacks, and Hispanics (%)

Age	White	White men	White women	Black	Black men	Black women	Latino	Latino men	Latino women
65 years and over	8.9	6.5	10.8	22.4	17.1	25.8	18.8	17.6	19.6
65–74 years	7.6	6.3	8.7	19.4	13.3	23.5	18.9	20.1	18.0
75 years and over	10.4	6.7	12.9	26.4	22.4	29.1	18.5	13.1	21.8

Source: Adapted from U.S. Census Bureau, 2001.

The picture of the Latino population in 2000 can easily change. The factors that shape these changes are both internal to the United States and internal to the countries from which many Latinos come. The economy of the United States and the political situation and economic conditions of many Central and South American countries, as well as Puerto Rico, encourages many Latinos to leave their native land.

Although this "push–pull" description has validity in describing immigration processes, the Latino population of the United States also has a large component of individuals whose families have lived on their lands for many generations. This is particularly true of Latinos in New Mexico. By 1988, a study by the National Hispanic Council on Aging revealed that a substantial proportion of the older Latino respondents were fifth-generation Americans (Sotomayor & Curiel, 1988).

Latinos are becoming more represented in all parts of the country, but the largest percentage (44.7%) live in the western United States. The Latino population in that part of the country is predominantly Mexican. Cubans are the predominant Latino population in Florida, but, in New York, Puerto Ricans are the predominant Latino population (U.S. Census Bureau, 2001).

A concentrated population has obvious implications for political change, and these changes are beginning to appear. Latino politicians now hold major state and national political offices. In the past, the growth of political power on the part of Latinos was slow, because of their low participation at the polls (Torres-Gil, 1986). Increasing numbers of Latinos are becoming U.S. citizens, and, as the numbers of Latino voters continue to grow, the efforts of politicians to woo this vote are increasingly apparent.

Economic Status and Education

Despite their newly realized political power, the current economic situation of Latinos in the United States is not positive. In 2001, 21% of all Latinos were living below the poverty level (Pear, 2002). This negative situation extends to the Latino elderly. As is true among Blacks, poverty rates among Latino elderly are substantially higher than those for Whites (Table 3.1).

Among Latinos over the age of 25, in 2000, 57% had graduated from high school. This figure is negative in comparison with the much larger percentage (88.4%) of Whites who had completed high school. Importantly, 27.3% of Latinos over age 25 had less than a ninth-grade education, in comparison to only 4.2% of Whites. Because of the number of Latino groups now represented in the United States, there is diversity in their educational backgrounds. An example is the fact that, although only 51% of Mexicans have completed high school, the proportion rises to 73% among Cubans (U.S. Census Bureau, 2001b). An ominous fact for future cohorts of Latino elderly is that, in 1998, about one third of Latino high school students were dropping out prior to graduation (Palen, 2001).

Age Distribution

The obvious economic needs of the Latino elderly have been given less attention than the needs of Latino youth, because Latinos remain a young population. In 2000, 36% of the Latino population was under age 18. Although the proportion of the population under age 18 has declined during the 1990s, it still remains larger than the 23.5% of the White population who are in this age category. The Latino population over the age of 65 now represents 5.3% of the total, but this is much less than the 14% of the White population (U.S. Census Bureau, 2001b). As was true of their educational status, a much higher proportion of Cubans are over the age of 65 (21%). Some of these older people were part of the initial wave of Cuban immigrants who fled the island after Fidel Castro came to power in 1960. The future age distribution of the Latino population in the United States will depend both on birth rates and immigration patterns. The 30.6% of the Latino population that has five or more family members is indicative perhaps of more extended family households, but also of higher birth rates. If fertility rates among Latinos decline, the proportion of older Latinos will continue to grow. Their representation in the Latino community will also be affected by immigration flows, since immigrants are usually younger individuals seeking not only political freedom, but also economic opportunities. A slowdown in immigration of Latinos to the United States would be indicated in a reduction in the current figure of 39.1% who are foreign-born (U.S. Census Bureau, 2001b).

Health Conditions

Unskilled jobs, low educational background, and low income are characteristics often related to poor health. Utilizing three data sets, Bastida and Gonzalez (1993) compared the health status of Mexican Americans and Whites in Texas to Puerto Ricans living in Connecticut. Not surprisingly, there were contrasting results: 75% of the Mexican American and Puerto Rican respondents rated their health as "fair" or "poor," compared to only 33% of the White elderly.

In 1998, Latinos had higher mortality rates from diabetes, homicide, liver disease, and HIV infection than did Whites. Higher mortality rates from these diseases, in part, may stem from health conditions, alcohol abuse, community problems, and inadequate health care. Age-adjusted rates among Latinos for heart disease and cancer, however, were lower than for the total population, Whites, or African Americans (Carter-Pokras & Zambrana, 2001).

The rates of the three most common forms of cancer (lung, breast, and prostate) are lower among Latinos than other groups. Cervical cancer, however, is found among Latino women at a rate that is 1.5 times higher than it is among Whites. Latinos also have a higher rate of some other forms of cancer (stomach, liver, esophagus, pancreas, and gallbladder). Latino women are more obese than the overall population and have a higher incidence of cardiovascular and cerebrovascular diseases (Villa & Torres-Gil, 2001). The reported incidence of diabetes is also almost twice as high among Latinos than it is among Whites (5.7 per 1,000 vs. 3.0 per 1,000) (Carter-Pokras & Zambrana, 2001). Diabetes rates among Latinos in the United States have been higher than those for heart disease.

Functional Status of Latino Elderly

Given the low-income, unskilled, and physically demanding jobs of Latinos in the United States, it is not surprising that their functional status is reported as lower than that of Whites. In a 1998 report, 40% of Medicare beneficiaries from Latino backgrounds reported difficulty performing at least one of the activities of daily living (ADLs) or instrumental activities of daily living (IADLs) (Olin & Liu, 1988). Many older Latinos may not be eligible for Medicare because they did not fulfill the eligibility requirements for this program or, as undocumented workers, had employment arrangements that did not include their involvement in Medicare and Social Security programs. Therefore, the Medicare data probably underestimates the extent of functional limitations among older Latinos.

Research attempting to compare the functional limitations of older Latinos with Whites or Blacks has not produced consistent results. In some cases, Latinos have been found to have more functional limitations than Blacks, but not more than Whites. Other studies have found Latinos to be significantly more limited than Whites (Carrasquillo, Lantigua, & Shea, 2000). In New York, older Latinos were found to be more functionally limited than Blacks, but these differences disappeared when the data were controlled for income and educational attainment (Berkman & Gurland, 1998). An analysis of national data reported similar functional limitations among non-Latino Whites and Latinos (Carrasquillo et al., 2000). There was also no difference in ability to carry out the ADLs between Latinos and Whites, in a major study completed in the San Luis Valley area of Colorado (Baxter, Bryant, Scarbo, & Shettlerly, 2001).

NATIVE AMERICAN AGED

Data Problems

Discussion of the Native American elderly is more difficult than any other minority group. The greatest problem is the lack of solid information. Perhaps because of their small numbers, public information often fails to include or provide separate information about Native Americans. Research on Native American elderly has been limited. John (1997) has also argued that the racial misclassifications of many Native Americans as White raises questions about the accuracy of much of the available health data, particularly data on death rates.

Currently, there are more than 500 recognized Native American tribes in the United States. Recognition as a tribe endows the tribe with eligibility for federal government programs. In terms of describing the Native American elderly, however, the important fact is that those Native Americans who do not belong to recognized tribal groups may not be counted in official statistics. On the 2000 census, 4.1 million people identified themselves as American Indian and Alaskan Natives, or some combination of these two categories with one or more other races. Of this 4.1 million, 2.5 million classified themselves as American Indian/Alaskan Native alone. Although they were forcibly dispersed into many states, Cherokees are the largest tribe (730,000 members), followed by Navajos (298,000). Among individuals who identified themselves as Native American alone, the population has grown 26% since the 1990 census. Adding together the population who identified themselves as Native American alone and American Indian with some other ethnic category, results in an increase of 110% in the Native American population since 1990 (U.S. Census Bureau, 2002a).

A greater willingness to be identified as Native American helps to account for the increase in Native American population in a number of states. In 2000, the largest numbers of Native Americans were living in California, followed by Oklahoma. An additional nine states had Native American and Alaskan Native populations of more than 100,000 people: Arizona, Texas, New Mexico, New York, Washington, North Carolina, Michigan, Alaska, and Florida. New York and Los Angeles were the cities with the largest number of Native American and Alaskan Natives (U.S. Census Bureau, 2001a). The largest numbers of Native Americans live in the western part of the United States (43%).

A distinction also needs to be made between Native Americans living on or off reservations. Native Americans in recognized tribes, living on or near reservation lands, are eligible for a variety of government programs and benefits. Once they move away from a reservation, programs targeted at Native Americans are not usually available. This distinction is particularly crucial in terms of the availability of heath care for the elderly.

The movement by Native Americans into urban areas increased during the 1980s. In 1970, rural areas accounted for more Native American residents than urban areas, in the 10 states with the largest Native American population. By 1991, the situation had changed, and the majority of Native Americans were living in urban areas in these states. Overall, 25% of Native Americans lived on reservations, and about 36% and 37%, respectively, resided in rural and urban areas (Hillabrant, Romano, Stang, & Charleston, 1991). A return to the reservation can resolve some split-family issues and result in an "economically efficient life career strategy" (Weibel-Orlando, 1988) for older American Indians. Among the elderly in Los Angeles, however, 61% planned to remain in the urban area (Weibel-Orlando & Kramer, 1989).

These findings do not confirm earlier research, in which American Indians indicated that they regarded their move to urban areas as temporary (Guillemin, 1975). A study comparing urban and reservation Native American elderly found problems of money, transportation, and social isolation were stressed by urban-based elderly Native Americans more often than by those living on the reservation (Manson, 1984). For a number of problems, urban Native American elderly reported fewer available social resources. The current status of Native Americans reflects the wavering and historically discriminatory policies of the American government.

Policies Toward Native Americans

In 1887, the Dawes-Severalty Act disbanded the tribes as legal entities entitled to hold land. Acreage on the reservations was distributed among families. In 25 years, these families would become owners of the properties. Many Native Americans, unused to intensive farming, were unable to survive farming their property and sold it to Whites before the 25 years had passed. These Indians then became dependent on government assistance. The Dawes Act was finally repealed in 1934. Its replacement was the Indian Reorganization Act, which aimed to make the reservations more self-sufficient in resources, education, and business opportunities. In the 1950s, the federal approach again shifted. Emphasis was placed on termination of the relationship between the government and the tribes. Native Americans were encouraged to move off reservations and into urban society. Some who left for the cities were able to find jobs as steelworkers or high-girder iron workers. Others, finding the urban culture totally alien, began to experience a variety of financial and mental health difficulties.

Each of these historical changes violated important aspects of Native American culture. Whites were not prepared to leave Native American traditions intact. Settling in one area was contrary to the living patterns of some tribes, but a nomadic pattern of life could not easily fit into a dominant culture that placed great emphasis on the concept of ownership of land and the inalienable right of the owner to use property in any way they wished. Settled tribes held the opposite view, that land was communal property. Unsuccessful in attempts to destroy Native Americans by force, the attitudes of non-Indian administrators on the reservation have usually been to enforce assimilation. As MacGregor describes the process:

> Children were virtually kidnapped to force them into government schools, their hair was cut, and their Indian clothes were thrown away. They were forbidden to speak in their own language. Life in the school was under military discipline, and rules were reinforced by capital punishment. Those who persisted in clinging to their old ways and those who ran away and were recaptured were thrown in jail. Parents who objected were also jailed. Where possible, children were kept in school year after year to avoid the influence of their families. (MacGregor, cited in Simpson & Yinger, 1965, p. 145)

The 1970s, 1980s, and 1990s have seen both the development of a change in American society toward Native Americans and the reassertion by tribal groups of their cultural backgrounds and treaty rights. This reassertion is manifested in such major arenas as the legal claims for land deeded to tribes as part of agreements with the American government. Popular movies and books have fostered new respect for Native American culture and crafts. Combining this reassertion of ethnic identity with improved social and economic conditions is the major challenge facing Native American groups.

The Impact of Aging

As is true of the other minority groups discussed in this chapter, the effects of aging occur early among Native Americans. High unemployment rates are one key indicator of problems that can have a major impact among younger Native Americans as they grow older. In areas where the Bureau of Indian Affairs is active, 16% of men and 13% of women over the age of 16 were unemployed in 1990, compared to 6.4% and 6.2% rates for men and women among the overall U.S. population (Indian Health Service, n.d.). Conditions such as these are a reason that, in 1981, research staff of the National Indian Council on Aging argued that conditions among rural Native Americans are so severe that, by age 45, this population is comparable to non-Indians over age 65, whom they studied in Cleveland (National Indian Council on Aging, 1981).

In 2000, 125,000 Native Americans and Alaskan Natives were over the age of 65. By 2050, this population is projected to grow to 530,000. This increase is dramatic, but Native Americans and Alaskan Natives will still only account for less than 1% of all older persons in the United States. The school-age population among Native Americans is increasing dramatically, but the overall population is aging (Hillabrant et al., 1991). The 1990 census indicated that the birthrate among Native Americans was 63% higher than it was for the overall U.S. population (Indian Health Service, n.d.). The net result of this high birth rate is there are more younger people and fewer older people among Native Americans. In 2000, only 6.3% of Native Americans were over age 65 (U.S. Census Bureau, 2001c), compared to a figure of 12.4% in the American population.

Socioeconomic Conditions

National data on income levels among Native Americans remains limited. The Census Bureau estimates that, between 1998 and 2000, the average poverty rate for all Native Americans was 26%. This rate is higher than the figures for Whites, Blacks, and Latinos (U.S. Census Bureau, 2001d). In 1990, the Census Bureau found that 36% of all Native Americans over age 65 were living below the poverty level (cited in Chapleski, 1997). Among the Native American populations served by the Indian Health Service, only 65% of the men and women over the age of 25, in 1990, had completed high school, compared to 75% of the overall U.S. population. The discrepancies are greater at the college level: 20% of the U.S. population had at least a Bachelor's degree, but this was true of only 9% of Native Americans (Indian Health Service, n.d.).

Health Problems and Mortality

Three of the 10 leading causes of death among Native Americans should be noted: (1) Chronic liver disease and cirrhosis is the sixth most common cause of death; (2) suicide is the ninth leading cause of death, and (3) homicide is the tenth (Anderson, 2001). These mortality figures can be related to poor living conditions, poverty, and alcohol abuse. Alcohol abuse is also manifest in other indices. In New Mexico, Native Americans were 8 times more likely to die from pedestrian–motor vehicle crashes, and were 30 times more likely to die from hypothermia. An analysis of these deaths (Gallaher, Fleming, Berger, & Seweil, 1992) indicates that 90% of the victims were intoxicated.

Native American elderly also evidence higher rates of a number of chronic illnesses than other populations. These include diabetes, liver and kidney disease, hypertension, arthritis, emphysema, and gallbladder problems (Chapleski, 1997). Type II diabetes is a problem that is affecting Americans in increasing numbers as a sedentary lifestyle and obesity become more common. Among Native Americans and Alaskan Natives who are part of the Indian Health Service population, the prevalence of diabetes increased by 29% between 1990 and 1997. Prevalence rates are higher among women, but, during this period, men evidenced a greater increase in diabetes rates than women. The age cohort with the highest prevalence of diabetes was Natives Americans between 45 and 64. Individuals over the age of 65 had the third highest rate of diabetes (24%). Between 1990 and 1997, diabetes rates increased 32% among Native Americans 45–64 and 25% among individuals 65 and over (Burrows, Geiss, Engelgau, & Acton, 2000).

Cancer rates are reported to be lower overall for Native Americans than for Whites, but there are variations according to tribe and geographic region in the United States. Breast, ovarian, prostate, and uterine cancer have lower prevalence rates among Native Americans (Rousseau, 1995). Given the prevalence of major health problems among older Native Americans, it is not surprising that only 18% of elders in 23 tribes described their health as "very good" or "excellent," compared to 31% of national samples (McDonald, 2001).

Life expectancy at birth has increased dramatically among Native Americans since the 1940s. In 1991, life expectancy at birth was 72.8 years for females and 64.9 years for males. This change has narrowed the gap between the life expectancy of Native Americans and Whites (John, 1997). Reexamining life expectancy data for undercounting or racial misclassification, Hahn and Eberhardt (1995) have calculated life expectancy at birth for Native American men in 1990 as 71 years and 78.7 years for women. At age 65, life expectancy was more than two years greater for Native American men than White men, with almost an equal difference between Native American and White women. As with Blacks, these figures indicate the operation of the crossover effect among older Native Americans.

In Oklahoma, a study of 60 Cherokee men and women between the ages of 55 and 87 found major limitations in physical functioning (McFall, Solomon, & Smith, 2000). In contrast, a sample of 309 Native Americans living in rural, urban, and reservation communities found that more than 70% of the sample had no problems with the ADLs and IADLs (Chapleski, Gelfand, & Pugh, 1997). A larger sample (2,705 elderly members of 27 tribes) found a range of limitations with ADLs. The largest proportion of problems was among the 31% of Native American elders who had difficulties in walking (McDonald, 2001).

ASIAN AGED

Asians in the United States

The history of Asians in the United States has been unique among the groups discussed in this chapter. During the early period of their arrival, Asians were seen as uneducated and docile workers who would work for cheap wages on sugar plantations in Hawaii, in the gold mining camps in California, or on the railroads under construction in the 1800s. Immigration restrictions, however, quickly arose, as nativist sentiment grew in the country. In 1882, the Chinese Exclusion Act was passed, closing off immigration to the United States from China. In many communities, Japanese workers were brought in to replace the Chinese. By 1900, there were 86,000 Japanese and 119,000 Chinese officially in the country. The year 1906 saw the first entrance of Filipinos into the United States, as workers in the territory of Hawaii. By 1985, Filipinos were almost equal in size to the Chinese American population, the largest Asian population in the United States.

In 1907, President Roosevelt signed an agreement with the Japanese government that ended Japanese immigration into the United States. The quota system instituted under the Johnson-Reed act in the 1920s did not include any Asian quotas. In 1941, Japanese Americans in California were shocked by their forced internment in camps. Internment resulted in their loss of land and businesses, and intense pressures on the family. This sad period in American history resulted in reparations being paid to former camp detainees in 1990.

The most recent immigration of Asians represents various groups of Southeast Asians displaced by the Vietnam War. In 1975, 125,000 Vietnamese arrived in the United States. By the middle of the 1980s, the number of refugees from all of Southeast Asia was approximately 800,000. The number of individuals attempting to leave Vietnam decreased in 1992. As Gardner, Robey, and Smith (1985) comment about Asian immigrants:

> These new residents are having an impact on this country that far exceeds their numbers, yet Americans know surprisingly little about them. As a group, Asian Americans do not resemble other racial or ethnic minorities. Less well-known is the fact that Asian Americans vary widely in their characteristics according to their cultural origins and when they arrived in the U.S. (p. 3)

More than 30 Asian groups are now represented in the U.S. population, including Chinese, Koreans, Indians, Pakistanis, Filipinos, Afghans, Hmong, Montagnards, Cambodians, Laotians, Thais, and Japanese.

During the 1990s, the Asian population grew from 2.8% of the total population to 4.2%. Five Asian groups (Chinese, Filipinos, Asian Indians, Vietnamese, and Koreans) now number over one million U.S. residents. Chinese and Filipinos remain the largest populations; Asian Indians and Vietnamese populations increased the most dramatically in the 1990s (by over 100% and 83% respectively) (Center for Urban Studies, 2002).

As is true of Latinos, Asians are concentrated in a number of states. The Asian population in California accounts for more than two thirds of the total Asian American population. An indication of the high representation of Asians in the western part of the United States is that

9.3% of all census respondents in that part of the country identified themselves wholly or in part as from Asian backgrounds. New York and Hawaii have the second- and third-largest Asian American populations in the 50 states (U.S. Census Bureau, 2002b). As is true of Latinos, Asian populations increased in many states during the 1990s. Maine was the only state in 2000 with a population that contained less than 1% Asian residents.

Age Distribution, Income, and Education

As the earliest immigrant groups to arrive from Asia, Japanese and Chinese have the largest number of older people. As the first Asian group to arrive in the United States with low birth rates, the Japanese American population declined 6% during the 1990s. This decline may be overstated, because of intermarriage rates that cause individuals with Japanese backgrounds to be listed as "other Asians" by the census (Center for Urban Studies, 2002). In 2000, poverty rates among Asian Americans were slightly higher than Whites (10.8% vs. 9.4%) and much lower than those of Blacks and Latinos (U.S. Census Bureau, 2001d).

Overall, Asian American elderly represented 2.3% of the total American population over the age of 65 (Administration on Aging, n.d.). Among Asian Americans, 7.3% were over the age of 65 (U.S. Census Bureau, 2000). The median age of Chinese and Japanese Americans was higher than the U.S. median in 1990, but the median age of the overall Asian American population in 2000 was approximately 3 years younger than the 35.3 years in the overall United States (U.S. Census Bureau, 2002b).

Generalizations about Asian elderly are difficult, not only because of their cultural diversity, but also because of the different patterns of immigration among these groups. The heyday of Japanese immigration to the United States was before the immigration restrictions of 1924 and after World War II. In contrast, Koreans entered the country primarily during the 1970s and 1980s, and Korean immigration began to decline dramatically in 1989 (Kim & Kim, 2001). The impact of this change can be seen in Table 3.2: Approximately half of all Korean Americans in 1998–2000 are foreign-born, but one fourth of Korean Americans are at least third-generation Americans. Over half of Japanese Americans are at least from third-generation backgrounds, and slightly less than half of Asian Indians fall into this category. Because of their major entrance into the country during the 1970s, less than 1% of all Vietnamese Americans are grandchildren of immigrants. What may surprise

TABLE 3.2 Nativity and Recency of Immigration of Asian Americans, 1990 and 1998–2000 (%)

	1990 foreign-born	1998–2000 foreign born	Second generation	Third and later generation
Asian total	66.8	49.2	23.7	27.1
Chinese	70.4	47.1	19.5	33.4
Filipinos	68.5	49.5	29.1	21.4
Japanese	35.2	22.7	22.2	55.2
Asian Indians	77.0	41.1	13.1	45.9
Koreans	82.2	52.4	21.9	25.7
Vietnamese	81.8	75.9	23.5	0.6
Other Asians	70.0	41.8	57.8	0.4

Source: Center for Urban Studies, 2000.

many Americans is that nearly one fourth of Vietnamese Americans are already second-generation individuals.

The educational background of older Asians varies among the groups and is in part related to their relative length of residence in the United States. Among Chinese, federal surveys indicate that 18.5% of Chinese males over age 65 had a college degree in 1981, compared to 10% of Whites. In contrast, only 6.8% of Chinese females, compared to 7.6% of White females, had completed college. Among individuals over age 25, however, there was a significantly larger proportion of Chinese than American Whites with no education (7.1% vs. 0.6%). Median household income of Chinese families was higher than that of Whites, a difference that may reflect a larger number of employed individuals in Chinese households (Yu, 1986). Among the total Asian American population, 39% over age 25 had completed four years of college in 1991. This figure is significantly higher than the 22% of Whites with college degrees (U.S. Census Bureau, 1992).

Health Status

For the most part, the health of Asian American elderly appears to be equivalent to, if not better than, that of other elderly groups. This would seem to be indicated by the long life expectancy at birth. Men born in 1990 had a life expectancy of 82 years and women 85.8 years. These life expectancies were at least 10 years greater than for White men and women. At age 65, Asian men and women had an average life expectancy that was at least five years greater than their White counterparts (Hahn & Eberhardt, 1995).

There are, however, differences in rates of particular health conditions among the different groups. Among Japanese Americans, diabetes and glucose intolerance is higher than among the White population. This problem is so marked that it has been estimated that 56% of Nisei children of Japanese immigrants have abnormal glucose tolerance. In general, the death rates for Chinese, Japanese, and Filipinos of all ages are lower than the comparable death rate for Whites. Among Asians, Japanese Americans have had the lowest death rates over the last 30 years.

An overall comparison of health characteristics of older Asian Americans and older Whites indicates reduced prevalence of hip fractures and coronary artery disease among older Asians. The incidence of liver, stomach, esophageal, and pancreatic cancers is higher among older Asians than Whites. There is also an increasing prevalence of diabetes among Japanese and Filipinos and increased prevalence of gout among Filipinos.

MENTAL HEALTH OF THE ETHNIC AGED

Although physical health issues are often the focus of discussions about the aging process, there are also important mental health issues that need to be examined. The compilation edited by Padgett (1995) provided a detailed summary of mental health issues among individual ethnic aged groups. Later studies confirm and add to the data provided in her volume.

Among older Americans, 12.3% are estimated to have mental health problems that require some intervention (Burns & Taube, 1990). The most important mental health problem among older person is depression. Depression can stem from a variety of sources. Older people suffering from serious illness may evidence a high level of depression. This comorbidity can be defined as the "co-occurrence of mental and physical illness" (Angel & Angel, 1995, p. 56). High levels of depression have been found among older Mexican Americans with diabetes, even when socioeconomic and demographic factors have been controlled (Black, 1999). Depressed individuals had more problems carrying out the varied ADLs than nondepressed individuals. In the Pacific Northwest, interviews have been conducted annually with older Native Americans, since 1984. As is true among Latinos, depression was related to low life satisfaction and problems carrying out the ADLs (Manson, 1995).

Although major chronic diseases can be related to depression, a number of other factors can be involved. Among older Latinos in Colorado, depression was also related to dissatisfaction with levels of social support, living alone, low income, and education. These factors, however, were the same for both older Latinos and Whites. The depression scores were substantially higher for Latino women than for White women, but there were no significant differences among men (Swenson, Baxter, Shetterly, & Hamman, 2000). Reviewing a number of studies completed from the 1970s through the mid-1990s, Mui (1996) reported similar results. Factors such as poor health and socioeconomic conditions, limited social support, and living alone figured as correlates of depression in many of the studies. In a number of the studies, depression was more common among women than men.

Severe depression can be related not only to difficulties in daily functioning. Depression has been noted as a major cause of suicide among Chinese immigrants (Mui, 1996). Among 150 older Chinese immigrants in Houston, feelings of grief and loss at leaving the home country were also found to be related to depression (Casado & Leung, 2001).

Besides depression, dementia (including Alzheimer's disease) is perhaps the most widely discussed mental health problem affecting older people. Comparing rates of dementia among the ethnic aged is still difficult, partly because dementia often goes unrecognized. An example is the high rates of unrecognized dementia found in a study of 191 noninstitutionalized older Japanese American men in Hawaii (Ross et al., 1997).

For immigrants, there are additional factors that can have a negative impact on their mental health. Many immigrants leave spouses, children, or other relatives behind, when they emigrate. Other immigrants find that their skills and backgrounds are not highly regarded in the new country, or that they cannot meet licensing requirements that allow them to practice their profession. For all immigrants, there is the problem of adapting to a new culture and, in many cases, the need to learn a new language. The discussion of the dilemmas faced by Haitian immigrants to the United States can be generalized to many older immigrants:

> The migration experience from Haiti to the United States has been more traumatic for some of the elderly because it subverted the natural rhythm of events that would have led to retirement. For these individuals, retirement began too early, as they were forced into a situation of dependency while in their early fifties. . . . This forced retirement was imposed on them not because they had reached an acceptable age to retire, had enough money to take care of themselves, did not want employment, or could not work due to chronic illness but because they were placed in a situation of withdrawal against their will. (Laguerre, 2001, p. 106)

Upon arrival in the new country, many immigrants may not immediately confront the emotional implications of immigration. Instead, their concentration may be on the primary needs of finding a place to live or a job. As the immigrant begins to acclimate to the new environment, some of the losses caused by the immigration process may surface, particularly the losses incurred by refugees who have left their homeland against their will. As Hao and Johnson (2000) note, immigrants vary in their ability to adapt to the demands of their new environment. Less resilient immigrants may never be able to recover from the losses encountered through migration, and may have poorer mental health. In their examination of factors that supported immigrants between the ages of 51 and 61, the presence of a spouse proved very important. Any discussion of mental health issues among the ethnic aged must therefore carefully distinguish between immigrants and natives. Berdes and Zych (1996) argue that immigrants "do not have access to the vital images of aging prevalent in American culture and they may simultaneously lack the family support structure in their culture of origin" (p. 58).

Zamanian et al. (1992) have examined the relationship between acculturation and depression. Using a broad definition of acculturation, the researchers found that more acculturated older Mexican Americans evidence lower levels of depression: "Our results imply that letting go of the Mexican culture in favor of the dominant (Anglo) culture may buffer one against depression" (Zamanian et al., 1992, p. 120). In this sense, it is not the inherent superiority of one culture over another that assists the older Mexican Americans. Bicultural or acculturated individuals are able to participate more fully in the larger society and not feel isolated, particularly if they do not live in a Latino community or have an extensive social support network (Zamanian et al., 1992).

This chapter has surveyed some of the major characteristics of various groups of ethnic aged in the United States. The obvious question that arises from this survey is: How can effective and adequate services be provided to groups that are so different? This question is the basis of the discussion in chapter 4.

REFERENCES

Administration on Aging. (n.d.). *Facts and figures: Statistical resources to effectively serve minority older persons.* Retrieved February 12, 2002, from *http://www.aoa.gov/ minorityaccess/stats.html*

Anderson, R. (2001). *National vital statistics reports. Deaths: Leading causes for 1999.* Retrieved April 15, 2002, from *http://www.cdc.gov/nchs/data/nvsr49/nvsr49_11.pdf*

Anderson, R., & DeTurk, P. (2002). *United States life tables, 1999: National vital statistics report.* Hyattsville, MD: National Center for Health Statistics.

Angel, R., & Angel, J. (1995). Mental and physical comorbidity among the elderly: The role of culture and social class. In D. Padgett (Ed.), *Handbook on ethnicity, aging and mental health* (pp. 47–72). Westport, CT: Greenwood.

Associated Press. (2002, September 13). Life expectancy nears 77 years. *New York Times,* A21.

Bastida, E., & Gonzalez, G. (1993). Ethnic variations in measurement of physical health status: Implications for long-term care. In C. Barresi & D. Stull (Eds.), *Ethnic elderly in long-term care* (pp. 22–36). New York: Springer Publishing.

Baxter, J., Bryant, L., Scarbro, S., & Shetterly, S. (2001). Patterns of rural Hispanic and Non-Hispanic White health care use: The San Luis Valley health and aging study. *Research on Aging, 23,* 37–60.

Berdes, C., & Zych, A. (1996). The quality of life of Polish immigrants and Polish American ethnic elderly. *Polish-American Studies, 53,* 17–43.

Berkman, C., & Gurland, B. (1998). The relationship between ethnoracial group and functional level in older persons. *Ethnicity and Health, 3,* 175–188.

Black, S. (1999). Increased health burden associated with comorbid depression in older diabetic Mexican Americans. *Diabetes Care, 22,* 56–64.

Burns, B., & Taube, C. (1990). Mental health services in general medical care and in nursing homes. In B. Fogel, A. Furino, & G. Gottlieb (Eds.), *Mental health policy for older Americans: Protecting minds at risk.* Washington, DC: American Psychiatric Press.

Burrows, N., Geiss, L., Engelgau, M., & Acton, K. (2000). Prevalence of diabetes among Native Americans and Alaskan Natives, 1990–1997. *Diabetes Care* (n.d). Retrieved April 15, 2002, from *http://www.findarticles.com/cf_0/m0CUH/12_23/68322723/p1/articlejhtml*

Carrasquillo, O., Lantigua, R., & Shea, S. (2000). Differences in functional status of Hispanic versus non-Hispanic elders: Data from the Medical Expenditure Panel Study. *Journal of Aging and Health, 12,* 342–361.

Carter-Pokras, O., & Zambrana, R. (2001). Latino health status. In M. Aguirre-Molina, C. Molina, & R. Zambrana (Eds.), *Health issues in the Latino community* (pp. 23–54). San Francisco: Jossey-Bass.

Casado, B., & Leung, P. (2001). Migratory grief and depression among elderly Chinese immigrants. *Journal of Gerontological Social Work, 36*(1/2), 5–26.

Center for Urban Studies. (2002). *Working paper 7: Asian in the United States, Michigan and metropolitan Detroit.* Detroit: Wayne State University Center for Urban Studies.

Chapleski, E. (1997). Long-term care among American Indians. In K. Markides & M. Miranda (Eds.), *Minorities, aging and health* (pp. 367–389). Thousand Oaks, CA: Sage.

Chapleski, E., Gelfand, D., & Pugh, K. (1997). Great Lakes American Indian elders and service utilization: Does residence matter? *Journal of Applied Gerontology, 16,* 333–354.

Dilworth-Anderson, P., Williams, I., & Williams, S. (2001). Urban elderly African Americans. In L. Olson (Ed.), *Age through ethnic lenses: Caring for the elderly in a multicultural society* (pp. 95–102). Lanham, MD: Rowman and Littlefield.

Federal Interagency Forum on Aging-Related Statistics. (2001). *Older Americans 2000: Key Indicators of Well-Being* (2000). Washington, DC: Author.

Ferris, M. (2000, November/December). Racial disparities in health care for the elderly. *Geriatric Times, 1*(4). Retrieved March 7, 2002, from *http://www.medinfosource.com/gt/2000/209html*

Foner, E. (1988). *Reconstruction: America's unfinished revolution.* New York: Harper and Row.

Gallaher, M., Fleming, D., Berger, L., & Sewell, M. (1992). Pedestrian and hypothermia deaths among Native Americans in New Mexico. *Journal of the American Medical Association, 267,* 1345–1348.

Gardner, R., Robey, B., & Smith, P. (1985). *Asian Americans: Growth, change and diversity.* Washington, DC: Population Reference Bureau.

Guillemin, J. (1975). *Urban renegades: The cultural strategies of American Indians.* New York: Columbia University Press.

Hahn, R., & Eberhardt, S. (1995). Life expectancy in four U.S. racial/ethnic populations: 1990. *Epidemiology, 6,* 352–356.

Hao, L., & Johnson, N. (2000). Economic, cultural and social origins and of well-being: Comparisons of immigrants and natives and mid-life. *Research on Aging, 22*, 599–629.

Hillabrant, W., Romano, M., Stang, D., & Charleston, M. (1991). *Native American education at a turning point: Current demographics and trends, 1991.* Washington, DC: Department of Education, Indian Nations at Risk Task Force.

Indian Health Service. (n.d.). *Trends in Health, 1998.* Retrieved April 18, 2002, from *http://www.his.gov/PublicInfo/publications/trends/98/*

Jackson, J. J., & Sellers, S. (2001). Health and the elderly. In R. Braithwaite & S. Taylor (Eds.), *Health issues in the Black community* (2nd ed.) (pp. 81–96). San Francisco: Jossey-Bass.

John, R. (1997). Aging and mortality among American Indians: Concerns about the reliability of a crucial indicator of health status. In K. Markides & M. Miranda (Eds.), *Minorities, aging and health* (pp. 79–99). Thousand Oaks, CA: Sage.

Johnson, H., Gibson, G., & Luckey, I. (1990). Health and social characteristics: Implications for services. In Z. Harel, E. McKinney, & M. Williams (Eds.), *Black aged: Understanding diversity and service needs* (pp. 113–121). Newbury Park, CA: Sage.

Jones, L., Hernandez-Valero, M., Esparza, A., & Wilson, D. (2001). Cancer. In R. Braithwaite & S. Taylor (Eds.), *Health issues in the Black community* (2nd ed.) (pp. 209–225). Francisco: Jossey-Bass.

Kim, S., & Kim, K. (2001). Intimacy at a distance, Korean American style. In L. Olson (Ed.), *Age through ethnic lenses: Caring for the elderly in a multicultural society* (pp. 45–58). Lanham, MD: Rowman and Littlefield.

Laguerre, M. (2001). Diasporic aging: Haitian Americans in New York City. In L. Olson (Ed.), *Age through ethnic Lenses: Caring for elderly in a multicultural society* (pp. 103–112). Lanham, MD: Rowman and Littlefield.

Manson, S. (1984). *Final report. Problematic life situations: Cross-cultural variation in support mobilization among the elderly.* Portland, OR: Institute on Aging: School of Urban and Public Affairs, Portland State University.

Manson, S. (1995). Mental health status and needs of the American Indian and Alaska Native elderly. In D. Padgett (Ed.), *Handbook on ethnicity, aging and mental health* (pp. 132–144). Westport, CT: Greenwood Press.

Manton, K. (1982). Differential life expectancy: Possible explanations during the later ages. In R. Manuel (Ed.), *Minority aging: Social and psychological issues* (pp. 63–70). Westport, CT: Greenwood Press.

McDonald, L. (2001). *Native American elders compared to the nation: A profile of needs.* Paper presented at the annual conference of the National Association of Area Agencies on Aging.

McFall, S., Solomon, J., & Smith, P. (2000). Health related quality of life in older Native American primary care patients. *Research on Aging, 22*, 692–714.

Mui, A. (1996). Depression among elderly Chinese immigrants: An exploratory study. *Journal of Gerontological Social Work, 30*, 147–166.

National Caucus and Center on Black Aged. (1989). *Health status of aged blacks.* Washington, DC: Author.

National Indian Council on Aging. (1981). *American Indian elderly: A national profile.* Albuquerque, NM: Author.

Olin, G., & Liu, H. (1998). *Health and health care of the Medicare population.* Rockville, MD: U.S. Department of Health and Human Services.

Padgett, D. (Ed.). (1995). *Handbook on ethnicity, aging and mental health.* Westport, CT: Greenwood Press.

Palen, J. (2001). *Social problems for the twenty-first century.* New York: McGraw-Hill.

Pear, R. (2002, September 25). Number of people living in poverty increases in U.S. *New York Times*, A1, A19.

Ross, G., Abbott, R., Petrovitch, H., Masaki, K., Murdaugh, C., Trockman, C., et al. (1997). Frequency and characteristics of silent dementia among elderly Japanese-American men: The Honolulu-Asia Aging Study. *Journal of the American Medical Association, 277*, 800–805.

Rousseau, P. (1995). Native-American elders: Health care status. *Clinics in Geriatric Medicine, 11*(1), 83–95.

Scheiner, S. (1974). The Negro at work: Blacks in Harlem, 1865–1920. In C. Greer (Ed.), *Divided society: The ethnic experience in America* (pp. 196–214). New York: Basic Books.

Simpson, G., & Yinger, G. (1965). *Racial and cultural minorities.* New York: Harper and Row.

Sotomayor, M., & Curiel, H. (1988). *Hispanic elderly: A cultural signature.* Edinburgh, TX: Pan American University Press.

Swenson, C., Baxter, J., Shetterly, S., & Hamman, R. (2000). Depressive symptoms in Hispanic and non-Hispanic white rural elderly: The San Luis Valley health and aging study. *American Journal of Epidemiology, 152*, 1048–1055.

Torres-Gil, F. (1986). The Latinization of a multigenerational population: Hispanics in an aging society. *Daedalus, 115*, 325–348.

U.S. Census Bureau. (1992). *The Asian and Pacific Islander population in the United States: March 1991 and 1990.* Washington, DC: U.S. Government Printing Office.

U.S. Census Bureau. (2000). *Asian and Pacific Islander population in the United States, March 2000 (update).* Retrieved June 25, 2002, from *http://www.census.gov/population/socdemo/race/api/ppl-146/tab01.txt*

U.S. Census Bureau. (2001a). *Census Bureau news: California, Oklahoma show largest American Indian and Alaskan Native population.* Retrieved January 13, 2002, from *http://www.census.gov/population/www/cen2000/briefs.html*

U.S. Census Bureau. (2001b). *Current Population Survey, March 2000.* Racial Statistics Branch, Population Division.

U.S. Census Bureau. (2001c). *General demographic characteristics by race for the U.S.: 2000.* Retrieved June 15, 2001, from *http://www.census.gov/population/cens2000/phc-t15/tab03.xls*

U.S. Census Bureau. (2001d). *Poverty in the United States: 2000.* Retrieved June 10, 2002, from *http://www.census.gov/prod/2001pubs/p60-214.pdf*

U.S. Census Bureau. (2002a). *American Indian and Alaskan Native population: Census 2000 brief.* Retrieved April 15, 2002, from *http://www.census.gov/prod/2002pubs/c2kbr01-15.pdf*

U.S. Census Bureau. (2002b). *The Asian population, 2000: Census 2000 brief.* Retrieved April 22, 2002, from *http://www.census.gov/prod/2002pubs/c2kbr01-16.pdf*

Villa, V., & Torres-Gil, F. (2001). The later years: The health of elderly Latinos. In M. Aguirre-Molina, C. Molina, & R. Zambrana (Eds.), *Health issues in the Latino community* (pp. 157–178). San Francisco: Jossey-Bass.

Weibel-Orlando, J. (1988). Indians, ethnicity as a resource and aging: You can go home again. *Journal of Cross-Cultural Gerontology, 3,* 323–348.

Weibel-Orlando, J., & Kramer, J. (1989). *Urban American Indian elders outreach project.* Los Angeles: Los Angeles County Area Agency on Agency, Department of Community and Senior Citizen Services.

Yu, E. (1986). Health of the Chinese elderly in America. *Research on Aging, 8,* 84–109.

Zamanian, K., Thackerey, M., Starrett, R., Brown, L., Lassman, D., & Blanchard, A. (1992). Acculturation and depression in Mexican-American elderly. *Clinical Gerontology, 11*(3/4), 109–121.

Chapter Four

Security and the Ethnic Elderly

The diversity of ethnic backgrounds among the American aged places special demands on service providers. Regardless of their discipline, providers must understand the ethnic backgrounds of older people, if they are to effectively deliver services. Many differences among ethnic groups need to be taken into consideration. This chapter examines basic factors that impinge on the older person's life. No attempt is made to grapple with the elusive concept of "successful aging." Instead, the discussion focuses on the security that ethnic aged persons have or need in their later years. For the purposes of this discussion, security is viewed as a multidimensional concept that includes financial security, health status, health care, and a sense of overall personal security. As is true of any issue that concerns the ethnic aged, security must be differentiated by age, as well as by immigration cohort.

AGE COHORT DIFFERENCES

In the field of aging, *age cohort* (individuals born at the same time) has proven to be a crucial analytical concept. All individuals born at the same time share similar life events. Obviously, persons born into poor families will have different experiences than children of rich parents. However, both groups encounter the same historical events that can shape attitudes over a lifetime. Their responses to these events may differ according to the resources available to each group.

Individuals who were 70 years old in 1990 were teenagers during the Great Depression of the 1930s. The depression had devastating consequences for millions of families and resulted in massive unemployment. The hardships of the depression years had an impact on attitudes about work and savings and the role of federal and local government. Individuals who suffered economically during the depression may always be nervous about major expenditures of income, fearing the possibility of another depression. Their savings and spending habits may vary drastically from those people who were born after World War II, when the economy appeared to be on an extended growth track.

Individuals growing up during the 1930s also developed important dietary and health patterns. As a result of new knowledge and altered norms, individuals may change their behaviors as they grow older. Unfortunately, these changes may occur too late to prevent them from entering their later years with health conditions that cannot be easily remedied.

Cohorts that came of age after World War II had greater opportunities for extensive education than their elders. The GI Bill helped a large number of veterans obtain a college education after the war, resulting in older individuals with higher income levels than earlier cohorts. An increase in socioeconomic status with each succeeding age cohort is desirable, but this unidirectional trend is not preordained. As already noted, social conditions in major urban areas may produce future cohorts of older African American and Latino men and women with less education and fewer assets than their predecessors.

Immigration Cohort Differences

Besides the importance of age cohort, the individual's cohort of immigration also has an impact on attitudes, values, and socioeconomic status. Individuals who lived in another country before coming to the United States are potentially quite different in their orientation than American-born individuals from the same ethnic group. These potential differences cut across a number of dimensions: educational background; occupational skills; and attitudes toward the family, values and traditions, governmental assistance, and the importance of ethnic history and customs.

Among current older age groups, there are substantial differences between Poles who arrived in the United States as refugees from Europe during the Second World War and their American-born age peers. Similar differences exist among older Russian Jews who arrived in the United States during the 1970s and American-born elderly from Russian Jewish backgrounds.

Underestimation of these differences created problems among social workers providing services to new Russian Jewish immigrants. Expecting the new immigrants to match past experiences with American-born Russian Jews, social workers were dismayed at the immigrants' behaviors. The immigrants demanded services, attempted to manipulate the workers, often lied, and even resorted to attempted bribery ("For Russian-Jews," 1983). As increasing numbers of workers reported this behavior, it became clear that the Russians were repeating behavior that had proven effective, and even necessary, for survival in the Soviet Union.

Having come of age in the Soviet system with its massive bureaucracy, the Russian immigrants identified all providers as government workers and failed to comprehend the concept of a voluntary agency. The repertoire of behaviors exhibited to American agencies was the same that was utilized in daily transactions with officials in Russia. The attitudes and behaviors of elderly American-born Jews were thus of limited assistance in understanding and serving the new Russian immigrants.

Although often viewed by Americans as an undifferentiated group fleeing their country after the fall of the South Vietnamese government, there were also significant differences among Vietnamese refugees. Vietnamese who arrived in the United States before 1975 were often from educated urban backgrounds, and had held important diplomatic or governmental positions in South Vietnam. The "boat people," who arrived after 1975, were primarily from lower socioeconomic groups, such as peasant farmers or fisherman from rural backgrounds. In the United States, there has been conflict between these two groups, based on long-standing political and class differences.

Socioeconomic differences within a group can be expected to increase among the second and third generations of immigrants (children and grandchildren of the original immigrants), as these later generations obtain more education and become more diverse in their occupations. Despite the economic losses that resulted from the loss of property and the forced internment in camps during the Second World War, these changes have occurred among Japanese Americans, as well as other ethnic groups.

Age and immigrant cohort differences are neglected. As noted in Chapter 1, efforts to describe the characteristics of an ethnic group usually portray the group's characteristics at one point in time. This portrayal may be accurate at the time it is drawn, but it fails to capture the changes that occur in the ethnic culture as it responds to conditions in the environment in which it is placed. Any update of the portrayal is difficult, because not all aspects of a culture change in response to the environment. Some traditional cultural beliefs and behaviors may be drastically transformed, while others remain constant. Even more complex is the situation in which behaviors of the ethnic group change, but beliefs and values do not. Amish farmers in Pennsylvania, for example, have modified their agricultural practices to take advantage of some modern equipment, but they have not modified their strong beliefs about the modern way of life.

Labeling groups as "traditional" or "modern" is not a solution to the problem of classifying change among ethnic groups. As Penning and Chappell (1987) have shown in a study of White ethnic elderly in Manitoba, a group that adheres to strong traditional values of kinship and family authority, such as Jews, may be the most modern in education and socioeconomic status. The abandonment or maintenance of traditional values can thus not be explained purely in terms of changes in a group's income or education. Maintenance or renunciation of traditional values must be viewed against the backdrop of the needs of the aged and whether the traditional values are able to meet those needs.

NEEDS OF THE ETHNIC AGED

In planning, a distinction is also often made between *needs* and *wants*. "A need is the value judgment that some group has a problem that can be solved" (McKillip, 1987, p. 10). *Wants* are goods or services for which people are willing to pay. If these items are important enough, they can become demands: "Something people are willing to march for" (McKillip, 1987, p. 16). What people want in terms of goods and services may be greater than what they actually need in order to survive. The balance between needs and wants is not easy to attain and brings us squarely to the question of how large or extensive the social welfare "safety net" should be. The ultimate answer to that question is based not only on the needs of many groups within the population of a country, but also on the philosophical and ideological attitudes of its citizens. In the United States, there have been major limits placed on the safety net, because of long-standing attitudes that individuals have the responsibility to provide for themselves and not depend on government assistance.

Without debating the appropriate size or elements of a safety net for the ethnic aged, we can, in this chapter, examine their needs related to four major areas: physical, financial, health, and personal security. These elements are basic for all older persons. The objective achievement of security and the subjective feeling of security are not always the same: This is apparent in newspaper accounts about older people who lived in poverty, but after death were found to have had substantial amounts of money.

Physical security implies a sense of confidence about one's place in the environment. Possessing this confidence, a person does not feel that physical movement may result in harm. Harm can result if the physical surroundings are inhospitable (e.g., buildings with too many stairs, high bathtub rims, high shelves, and high light switches). Outside the home, high steps on buses, high curbs, and poorly lit streets and signs may produce perceptions of an inhospitable environment.

The relative security or insecurity of the physical environment may be related to the older person's physical health. It is not easy to provide a physically secure and hospitable environment for an older person who is in poor health and has difficulty walking. Home construction and the urban environment show little sensitivity to the physical needs of older people. This lack of attention compounds the problems of older people attempting to maintain their independence.

Physical Security and the Home

The ethnic aged who settled in urban communities when they were young often lived in apartment complexes unsuited to their physical needs. Many of the apartment buildings were built during a period when an elevator was not part of the building code unless the building was over four stories high. Even in ethnic communities where private homes predominate, two-story houses become increasingly onerous for older persons with physical problems. Garden apartment complexes of two stories became popular after World War II. The upper levels of these complexes become difficult to reach as their tenants age.

The growth of the aging population in the United States is only beginning to have an impact on design and construction. Recent legislation, including the Americans with Disabilities Act, requires more thought about physical disability in building design. Deficits in physical security are easier to alleviate within, rather than outside, the home. Nonslip carpeting, chair rails, and grab bars in bathtubs are all simple alterations.

Physical Security Outside the Home

Easy mobility within the home, or ease in the transition from the home to outside through ramps rather than stairs, does not resolve the physical security issues facing the older person. They need to feel secure making trips to the store, visiting friends, and going to social engagements or to medical appointments. Wheelchair ramps can be used to negotiate high curbs. Kneeling buses, whose front end lowers to allow passengers to enter, relieves the obstacles posed by high stairs.

Providing a sense of security against crime is more difficult outside the home. For some older people, a fear of being attacked may be evident even inside the home. Window bars and multiple locks are the stereotypical image of many urban areas. A lack of physical security within the living environment can become a major psychological stressor for older persons who spend most of their time at home.

A feeling of unsafe streets may also cause the older person to restrict social involvement. Focus groups, conducted as part of a study of senior centers (Gelfand, Bechill, & Chester, 1990), revealed that, although some center participants desired evening activities, they were afraid to attend programs held at inner city centers. As nondrivers, many of the participants would also have to wait on the street for buses. Among Chaldeans (Iraqi Christians) living primarily in suburban Detroit, one third noted that "crime was somewhat of a problem in their area" (Sengstock, 1999, p. 87).

Perceived physical vulnerability is more common among older than younger age cohorts. Despite this sense of vulnerability, there is little evidence that older individuals are more the target of attacks or robberies than other age groups (Gelfand, 1993). The reality of the situation is not as important as the perception of insecurity that affects the older person's behavior. Streets that are perceived as unsafe seriously hamper the efforts of ethnic aged to maintain social contacts. The advantages of living in proximity to neighbors or friends from the same ethnic background disappear, if older individuals do not feel secure about venturing outside their home. McAdoo (1993) suggests that, by limiting their activities outside the home, African American elderly reduce "crime stress."

Over time, many ethnically homogeneous communities undergo a change, as new ethnic groups become residents. Many ethnic aged do not view this change as a pleasant increase in diversity, but as a threatening situation. New ethnic cultures, with different values and different living patterns, may provoke trepidation, among the older ethnic aged, about venturing outside, shopping, or going to their clubs.

Social Security

When asked about their most important needs, many older people respond that they need enough income to live without worry and good health to enjoy the money they have accumulated. Although many older people have a variety of income sources, Social Security is among the most essential. The positive and negative features of the American Social Security system are highlighted if the American system is compared to one with different regulations, such as the old-age pension in Australia.

In the United States, Social Security is earmarked for retired individuals over age 65. In Australia, the term *Social Security* refers to a whole variety of income maintenance programs, often subsumed under the term *the dole.* Income maintenance programs for the elderly are referred to as "the old-age pension."

The differences between the American system and the Australian system are not merely those of terminology. In the United States, Social Security refers to an income maintenance program that is funded through payments made by workers. These payments (in 2002, 7.65% of the first $84,900 earned) are matched by the employer (Social Security Administration, 2002a). Self-employed individuals contribute the total amount otherwise paid by the employee and employer. At the end of 2001, a total of $432 billion of Social Security benefits were paid to 45.9 million people (Social Security Administration, 2002b). No funds from so-called general revenues, such as income taxes, are used to fund Social Security benefits. In Australia, the old-age pension is paid totally out of general revenue funds, that is, workers do not pay into any special fund out of their earnings.

Beyond whether the system is contributory or noncontributory is the issue of how much an individual can collect. In Australia, the old-age pension is means tested and is reduced substantially if the individual has a high income. Only individuals with less than $100,000 in assets are eligible for the full old-age pension. The only other restrictive element in the Australian old-age pension is that the individual has to have been a resident of Australia for at least 10 years. In many cases, older individuals who come to Australia under the family provision of Australian immigration law have to be supported by their children until they live long enough in Australia to qualify for the old-age pension. In the United States, length of time contributing to the Social Security program, rather than length of residence, determines an individual's eligibility. Recent refugees from the Soviet Union or Vietnam have the same eligibility for Social Security as older Poles who arrived in the United States after World War II. Official eligibility, however, is not an equalizing characteristic in a program that bases its benefits on how much individuals have contributed to the system. Individuals who have only recently arrived in the United States are not likely to have contributed a great deal of money to Social Security. Many refugees come into the country and are forced to take low-paying jobs, because of a lack of job skills, problems in communicating, or because their professional credentials are not accepted in the United States. Engineers and doctors from foreign countries may have to accept relatively low-income jobs as their first employment in the country, because their degrees or licenses are not recognized. The amount of money these émigrés pay into the Social Security trust fund may be low, because of their low wages.

In order to be fully eligible for benefits, a person must contribute for 10 years (40 quarters) to the Social Security system, in order to collect benefits when they reach the age of eligibility. In 2002, a worker had to earn $870 in one quarter of the year, in order for this quarter to be counted toward eligibility. If the refugee arrives when they are 55, they may not accumulate enough quarters to be fully insured. Even if they contribute enough quarters, their benefits may be limited, because of the low salaries they earned during this work period. This is particularly true for women, since salaries for women are still significantly lower than those of men. Unskilled women also may work cleaning homes and apartments. Both these women and their employers may omit payments to the Social Security system.

Social Security and Financial Security

By 2001, Social Security had become essential for millions of retirees and their spouses. Despite its importance, reliance on Social Security, as the primary or only source of income, is more common among older women than other groups. Within this group of older women, African American and Latino elderly are the individuals most likely to depend on Social Security. Social Security was the only source of income for one third of all older Black men and women (National Council of La Raza, n.d.). Older Latinos are similar to Black elderly in their dependence on Social Security benefits for their income. For 33% of older Latinos in 1998, Social Security was their only source of income (National Council of La Raza, n.d.).

In 1999, the average yearly benefit for White retirees under Social Security was $9,630. The benefit for African American retirees was $7,771 and for Latinos $7,584 (National Council of La Raza, 2001). There are also maximum benefits that can be obtained from Social Security. In 2002, an individual could receive a maximum of $1,660 per month ($19,200 per year).

The Social Security benefits of minority men and women provide clear evidence that minority elderly will not be able to be active members of a consumer society, if they rely on Social Security as their major source of support. As Table 4.1 indicates, White, African American, and Latino elderly differ in the receipt of income from other sources besides Social Security. Although almost two thirds of White elderly have income from assets such as dividends and interest, this is true of only 29% of Black elderly. A smaller percentage of Black than White older persons also have income from pensions (Social Security Administration, 2000a).

Social Security rewards stable work patterns. Gibson (1987) finds that older age cohorts of African American elderly have had more continuous work patterns than younger African Americans. This pattern exists despite the educational advantages of the younger individuals. Discontinuous work patterns are rooted in the high unemployment rates of young African Americans. Carried into the future, they are ominous in their impact: "If nothing is done to ameliorate the situation, millions of young Blacks will be even more disadvantaged when they reach old age than the present cohort of older Blacks in regard to continuous labor forces participation" (Gibson, 1987, p. 237).

Because of poor health, many African American workers do not reach conventionally defined ages of retirement, but retire early because of

TABLE 4.1   Percentage Receiving Income from Major Sources, by Race and Latino Origin, 2000

Source of income	White	Black	Latino
Social Security	91	88	77
Asset income	63	29	28
Pensions	43	33	22
Earnings	23	19	19
Supplemental Security Income	3	10	16

Source: Social Security Administration, 2000a.

disability. These "unretired retired" may adopt the perspective of the disabled worker, feel powerless to control their own fate, feel less satisfied with life, and play a less active part in the community (Gibson, 1987). The unretired-retired African American older person, and future cohorts of older workers with discontinuous work patterns, will receive low Social Security benefits because of their work history. This last group also includes women who remain out of the labor force for a number of years to raise children. As a result of lower salaries and breaks in their years of work, female Social Security beneficiaries received an average payment of $756 in 2001. Male beneficiaries received an average of $985 per month (Social Security Administration, 2002b).

Supplemental Security Income

African American and Latino elderly comprise a large percentage of older persons receiving Supplemental Security Income (SSI). SSI is a program dedicated to providing basic income for poor aged, blind, and disabled individuals living independently. Individuals who receive low Social Security benefits can also receive SSI up to its allowed benefit levels, if they meet its eligibility requirements. SSI was instituted in 1974 as a way for the federal government to administer the Old Age Assistance program, which included assistance to the blind and disabled. The Old Age Assistance program was formerly administered by the individual states. The federal government assumed control over the program because of the wide variations in the payments made by the states to eligible individuals.

The SSI program generates better equity than the previous state-run efforts. In 1998, almost 2 million people over the age of 65 received SSI benefits. Of this number, 62% were White, 30% Black, 3% Native American, and 5.4% Asian. Separated from the category of White or Black, 16% of SSI recipients were classified as Latino. Older immigrants accounted for one third of older recipients by 1995 (National Center for Policy Analysis, 2001). For more than one third of all of the recipients in each of these groups, except for Asians, SSI comprised 100% of their income. Among Asian recipients, 26% depended on SSI benefits as their sole income (Social Security Administration, 2000b).

SSI benefits are not set at a standard that would enable older people to live above the poverty level. In 2002, the maximum for an individual was $545 a month. Almost all states supplement this amount. In the states offering only basic SSI, the addition of Food Stamps helps to provide older people with the means to buy groceries, but does not enable them to live above the federal poverty level.

Beyond the question of its adequacy is the issue of the restrictive eligibility requirements for SSI. These eligibility requirements place limits on the amount of assets an individual can have, including the value of their car, income, cash, and even furnishings. Despite the restrictive eligibility of SSI, in the 1980s, many older people were eligible but not receiving SSI. The 1987 amendments to the Older Americans Act (OAA) authorized special outreach efforts to increase the numbers of eligible older people receiving SSI. In 1990, the Social Security Administration awarded a number of demonstration grants to organizations proposing innovative approaches to SSI outreach efforts.

As already noted, the SSI program is dedicated to older persons living independently. When an individual moves into a nursing home, their SSI benefits cease. When they live with a relative, such as a child or with any caregiver, their benefits are reduced by one third. The logic for this reduction is that it does not cost as much for the older person to live with others as independently.

For some families, this reduction may not be onerous, but, for poorer families, this one-third reduction may create major difficulties in the provision of care needed by the older relative. Because African American, Latino, and Native American families have lower income levels than White families, reduction in SSI benefits when an older relative lives in the family's home is particularly damaging. The reduction discourages the maintenance of family traditions, which encourage family responsibility for care of the older person. Instead, the family feels penalized for assuming some major caregiving tasks.

HEALTH SECURITY

An individual who possesses health security feels prepared to respond to health problems as they arise. A sense of health security also includes confidence that, if health problems are beyond the individual's capability, adequate health care is available. Development of this sense of health security has at least five parts:

1. knowledge about health factors, which enables individuals to adjust their lifestyles to the physical changes that accompany aging
2. a willingness to adjust a lifestyle to accommodate the aging process and preserve health
3. knowledge of the health services available in the community

4. access to health facilities
5. attitudes that encourage the use of these health facilities

The net result of health security for older persons should be a positive health status, which does not, however, mean the absence of any health problems. Older persons expect to have aches and pains, and do not expect to feel like 18-year-olds when they wake up in the morning.

Medicare and Health Security

Since 1965, Medicare has attempted to ensure that older persons have adequate health care. Medicare is available to anyone eligible for Social Security. An eligible older person is automatically enrolled in Part A of Medicare, which covers hospitalization. Part B, which reimburses 80% of doctor's fees, requires that a person enroll at the time they file for their Social Security benefits. The basic fee for Part B is set by the federal government and deducted monthly from a beneficiary's Social Security check. If the individual does not enroll in Part B at the time they file for Social Security benefits, the monthly fee is higher. In 2002, the monthly fee for Part B of Medicare was $54. The enactment of Medicare ensured that most older people would receive adequate hospital care, particularly if their hospital stays are not lengthy. The basic cost to the older patient in 2002 for Part A was a $812 deductible.

Low-income elderly may not even be able to pay the basic Medicare deductible. If their income is low enough, these older persons can receive Medicaid to cover this expense. In fact, the federal government now requires that states "buy in" to Medicare for older persons whose incomes are too high for Medicaid, but are at the federal poverty level.

A further problem with Medicare is its complex reimbursement procedure. Physicians can elect whether to accept assignment for their Medicare patients, which means that the physician will abide by the Medicare decision about the appropriate fees to be paid for their services. If the physician does not accept assignment, Medicare will pay 80% of the cost of the service at their approved rate, and the physician obtains the remainder of their fee from the patient. Many patients do not understand the meaning of assignment or inquire of their physicians whether they are participating providers. The lack of understanding may be greater among ethnic aged whose mastery of English is limited.

Health Insurance and Security

Medicare is usually available only to people over age 65. Retirees who have not reached this age, and younger individuals, must rely on other forms of private health insurance. Available data does not separate individuals without health insurance according to their legal or illegal immigration status, but the health insurance coverage of native-born individuals may be compared with that of immigrants (Table 4.2). Among the 18–64-year-old population in 1998, 38% of immigrants and 16% native-born individuals had no health insurance. The same relationship between immigrants and native-born can be seen when examined by ethnic backgrounds. The percentage of uninsured individuals naturally declines among the older population, because of Medicare insurance, but there is still a small proportion (5%) of immigrants over the age of 65 without any health insurance (Center for Immigration Studies, 2000).

Examined by ethnic background, Latinos have the highest percentage of individuals who are uninsured. Regardless of whether they are Asian, Black, or Latino, immigrants or native-born, the presence of a significant population of individuals without health insurance has substantial negative implications. Even if the uninsured population obtains Medicare insurance when they reach 65, lack of health coverage during their earlier years may mean that they enter their later years with major chronic health problems that could have been prevented with earlier interventions.

Health Care Costs

The medical expenses absorbed by older people have continued to rise, despite the introduction of Medicare. Older people are paying, out-of-pocket, the same percentage of their income as they were before Medicare. Rising health care costs do not permit the older population to reduce their health care spending. Inflation in costs is attributable

TABLE 4.2   Uninsured Persons, by Immigration Status and Age (%)

	Immigrant	Native-Born
Age 18–64	37.9	16.9
Age 65 and over	5.0	0.7
Asian	22.7	14.4
Black	29.5	2.4
Latino	44.6	24.8

Source: Adapted from Center for Immigration Studies, 2000.

to the health care needs of a growing population of older people, the use of expensive technology to meet these needs, and increases in doctor's fees, hospital costs, and the costs of medication. On average, older individuals were spending 19% of their income on health care (Crystal, Johnson, Harman, Sambamoorth, & Kumar, 2000). Unfortunately, older individuals in the lowest 20% income brackets spent 32% of their income for health care. In contrast, individuals in the top 15% income brackets spent 9% their income on health care.

Many older people have private "Medigap" policies to supplement their Medicare insurance, which closes the gap between what Medicare reimburses and their own expenses. These policies are too expensive for many ethnic aged. A lack of insurance that makes health care affordable and the unavailability of adequate health care are also often mentioned as underlying factors in differential mortality rates from diseases.

Many women may view health examinations as needed only when serious illness is detected, rather than as a preventive strategy. Pap smears, mammograms, and other techniques are important early detection techniques. A lack of insurance reimbursement reinforces low utilization of these screening tools. As the cost effectiveness of early detection becomes increasingly clear, Medicare has expanded its coverage to reimburse procedures such as Pap tests and mammograms. The task now is to convince older women, who do not see any symptoms of health problems, of the importance of these tests.

Among older men, the same need exists for better access and possible alterations in attitudes about health prevention. Deaths from colon cancer are higher among African American men aged 65 to 74 than among White men in the same age cohort, despite the treatability of this form of cancer when detected at an early stage.

PERSONAL SECURITY

The concept of *personal security* is not common in the gerontological literature and is difficult to define. Reker and Wong (1988) discuss personal meaning in one's life and what constitutes personal meaning. Their "fundamental postulate" is that "every individual is motivated to seek and to find personal meaning in human existence" (p. 238).

Personal meaning is part of personal security. An individual who is personally secure has a sense of stability about their life and a sense of certainty about status and roles. The components of personal security are a stable set of social relationships, which includes a social network for basic interaction, and a social support system that can be called upon for assistance. It is not possible to assert how many people must belong to the social network or be able and willing to provide assistance. Some older persons will perceive a small network as adequate. For others, only a large network that maintains a high frequency of contact will be sufficient to provide a sense of personal security.

Role Changes and Personal Security

Extensive role changes may diminish the individual's sense of personal security. Role changes are intrinsic to the life cycle. The question is, Do individual role changes reflect choices among alternatives, or are they forced upon the individual? Role changes that involve a major loss of roles are often imposed on ethnic aged who have limited education, lack of fluency in English, or problems in physical mobility. Role changes that displace traditional roles associated with older persons can also create problems.

In the United States, as in many contemporary industrialized societies, there is a lack of well-defined roles into which the older person can move. If the older person grew up in a society in which roles for the elderly are clearly defined, the move to American society, with its lack of distinct roles for the older person, may be disheartening. The new roles available to them may be ill-defined and offer only limited prestige. Replacement of traditional roles is often possible for the ethnic aged, but these new roles may not be to their liking. A primary role for many ethnic aged is child care. In many ethnic families, the provision of child care by the older person is crucial in allowing family members to work. The problem for the older ethnic aged person lies not in their assumption of child care provision, but in the fact that child care often becomes their only role.

A shift in roles of this nature is revealed in a study of older Salvadorans in the Washington, DC, area (Gelfand, 1989). In El Salvador, the roles of these respondents included teaching their children and giving advice. In the United States, these roles had been replaced by child care. Decision-making responsibilities were difficult for the older Salvadorans to undertake, because they were not familiar enough with American culture.

Many traditional ethnic communities stress the wisdom of, and respect for, the elderly. But an inability to speak English, and a lack of knowledge of urban customs and occupations, has denigrated the traditional role of many Asian elderly in family decision-making. The result is a loss of respect from children (Min, 1988).

Role Changes and Rituals

Major shifts in roles associated with age changes are recognized in many cultures through prescribed rituals and ceremonies. As Keith notes (1990), in the United States, few rituals are attached to life stage and role changes. Employed persons usually are given a party upon their retirement. This party represents the separation aspect of a rite of passage, but the reincorporation of the older person into new roles through ritual is lacking.

For the ethnic aged who have spent their life in the United States, traditional rites of passage that defined new roles for the older person may have been long foregone. In some cases, the ritual may be retained as a symbolic gesture, without real impact on the daily life of the older person.

An interesting example of the maintenance of a ritual with altered meaning is the *kankrei* among Nisei (second-generation Japanese Americans born between 1915 and 1935) (Doi, 1991). In traditional Japanese culture, the *kankrei* is observed primarily for men. The ritual celebrated the man's retirement from work and from the responsibilities of middle age. The adult children were handed responsibility for control of the farm and the household. In return, the older individual was allowed new freedoms, including "swearing, sexual joking, and lewd dancing" (Doi, 1991, p. 155)

The celebration of the *kankrei* among Japanese American families is usually initiated by the Sansei (third-generation) children as a surprise party, and has become part of the 60th birthday celebration. Some of the elements of the traditional ritual, such as dress, are included in the party, as are elements of American birthday celebrations, such as a birthday cake. Most importantly, the *kankrei* celebrations among Japanese American families carry no special import related to role changes for the 60-year-old person:

> They [the 60-year-old Nisei] are being celebrated with a Japanese ritual, yet they know they are not Japanese. They are being ushered into old age, yet they are not old. They provided care to aging Issei parents yet cannot expect and say they do not want the same from their children. And they will be old soon in an American setting that devalues the elderly. (Doi, 1991, p. 161)

The *kankrei* is one way that the Nisei address their aging, and it also indicates the responsibility and coming of age of the Sansei.

In Los Angeles, there has been a revived interest in El Dia de los Muertos (the Day of the Dead) among Latinos. Similar to the Catholic All Saint's Day, this ritual ceremony recognizes ancestors and honors older persons. Cordero-Aranda (1989) emphasizes the therapeutic functions of this ritual ceremony. The ceremony allows older Mexican Americans to maintain the symbols of their culture. In addition, the observance of El Dia de los Muertos brings the family together and reinforces family cohesion.

Achieving Personal Security

Rapid changes in life situation would seem to threaten personal security. The death of a spouse, or loss of a job because of retirement, can be destabilizing events, which may result in the widow or widower adopting different roles. In addition, the older person may relocate and leave a residence that they have occupied for many years and that has significant personal meaning.

Fortunately, not all life changes have a negative impact. Many older people view retirement as a desired outcome, because of boredom with their job. Retirement offers a chance to undertake new projects. For less-affluent older persons, retirement may represent a release from demanding physical labor. These types of differences were evident among White, African American, and Latino elderly in California, who were asked during the 1970s about what they expected from retirement. The responses varied along ethnic lines, but the three groups also varied significantly in occupational status (Ragan & Simonin, 1978).

Even as tragic an event as the death of a spouse opens up possibilities for the marital survivor. The new widow or widower finds an opportunity to rethink how to spend their time. They may begin to engage in new activities, particularly if they previously had been heavily involved in caregiving for the deceased spouse. This new engagement may provide a sense of purpose crucial to their self-esteem after many years of sharing their lives with a partner. Indeed, the new activities may provide the older person with a greater sense of meaning than they had in earlier years. By linking the widow or widower with a new, and perhaps larger social network, involvement in activities may reinforce the older person's sense of personal security.

Financial, physical health, and personal security are all components of a total sense of security on the part of the older person. The relationships among these various forms of security are not additive, that is, financial plus physical, plus health, plus personal security does not necessarily provide overall security. A lack of financial security may be offset for one older person by a high level of personal security. The same compensatory mechanism may occur among older persons lacking other types of security.

An ethnic culture offers a variety of activities for the older person, as well as a patterned set of stable relationships among family, friends, and in a geographic area. These relationships can provide the personal security desired by the older person. The role of the family in the development of a sense of security extends beyond its social interactions, into the arena of actual assistance to the older person. The role of the family and another major institution, the church, in assisting the ethnic aged, is examined in Chapter 5.

REFERENCES

Center for Immigration Studies. (2000). *Without coverage: Immigration's impact on the size and growth of the population.* Retrieved May 3, 2002, from *http://www.cis.org/articles/2000/coverage/findings-cont.html*

Cordero-Aranda, M. (1989). El Dia de los Muerto: A spiritual link for better mental health. *The Aging Connection, 10*(5), 13.

Crystal, S., Johnson, R., Harman, J., Sambamoorth, S., & Kumar, R. (2000). Out-of-pocket health care costs among older Americans. *Journal of Gerontology: Social Sciences,* S41–50.

Doi, M. (1991). A transformation of ritual: The Nisei 60th birthday. *Journal of Cross-Cultural Gerontology, 6,* 153–161.

For Russian-Jews, a restoral of faith. (1983). *Practice Digest, 5,* 13–16.

Gelfand, D. (1989). Immigration, aging and intergenerational relationships. *The Gerontologist, 29,* 366–372.

Gelfand, D. (1993). *The aging network* (4th ed.). New York: Springer Publishing.

Gelfand, D., Bechill, W., & Chester, R. (1990). *Maryland senior centers: Programs, services and linkages.* Baltimore: School of Social Work, University of Maryland at Baltimore.

Gibson, R. (1987). Defining retirement for Black Americans. In D. Gelfand & C. Barresi (Eds.), *Ethnic dimensions of aging* (pp. 224–238). New York: Springer Publishing.

Keith, J. (1990). Age in social and cultural context. In R. Binstock & L. George (Eds.), *Handbook of aging and the social sciences* (pp. 91–105). San Diego: Academic Press.

McAdoo, J. (1993). Crime, stress, self-esteem and life satisfaction. In J. Jackson, L. Chatters, & R. Taylor (Eds.), *Aging in Black America* (pp. 38–48). Newbury Park, CA: Sage

McKillip, J. (1987). *Need analysis: Tools for the human services and education.* Newbury Park: CA: Sage.

Min, P. G. (1988). The Korean American family. In C. Mindel, R. Habenstein, & R. Wright, Jr. (Eds.), *Ethnic families in America: Patterns and variations* (3rd ed.) (pp. 210–230). New York: Elsevier.

National Center for Policy Analysis. (2001). Immigration issues: Welfare attracts elderly immigrants. Retrieved January 5, 2002, *from http://ncpa.org/pd/immigrat/pdimm16.html*

National Council of La Raza (n.d.). *Hispanic retirement fact sheet.* Retrieved March 20, 2002, from *http://www.nclr.org/policy/socialsecurity*

National Council of La Raza. (2001). Issue brief Number 5. *Financial insecurity amid growing wealth: Why healthier savings is essential to Latino prosperity.* Retrieved May 2, 2002, from *http://www.nclr.org/policy/briefs/Issue%20Brief%205.pdf*

Penning, M., & Chappell, N. (1987). Ethnicity and informal supports among older adults. *Journal of Aging Studies, 1,* 125–160.

Ragan, P., & Simonin, M. (1978). *Social and cultural contexts of aging, community survey report.* Los Angeles: University of Southern California, Andrus Gerontology Center.

Reker, G., & Wong, P. (1988). Aging and an individual process: Towards a theory of personal meaning. In J. Birren & V. Bengtson (Eds.), *Emergent theories of aging* (pp. 214–246). New York: Springer Publishing.

Sengstock, M. (1999). *Chaldean Americans: Changing conceptions of American identity.* New York: Center for Migration Studies.

Social Security Administration. (2000a). *Income of the aged chartbook, 2000.* Retrieved June 30, 2002, from *http://www.ssa.gov.statistics/income_aged/2000/iac00.html*

Social Security Administration. (2000b). *SSI annual statistical report.* Retrieved May 2, 2002, from *http://ssa.gov/statistics/ssi_annual_stat/2000/sect2.html#top*

Social Security Administration. (2002a). *Facts and figures about Social Security.* Retrieved June 30, 2002, from *http://ssa.gov/statistics/fast_facts/2002/ff2002html#generalinfo*

Social Security Administration. (2002b). *2002 OASDI annual report.* Retrieved May 4, 2002, from *http://www.ssa.gov/OACT/TR/TR02/III_fyoper.htm#8458*

Chapter Five

Family and Religious Organizations as Sources of Assistance

The family and religious organizations can be important elements in meeting the needs of an aging population. Major variations in cultural attitudes regarding these social institutions are examined in this chapter. Migration and relocation, however, can dramatically alter the profile of the family and the influence of traditional religious organizations. Immigration from another country to the United States is discussed in Chapter 2. The impact of internal migration of the ethnic aged also needs to be evaluated.

PATTERNS OF INTERNAL MIGRATION

Factors in Internal Migration

Litwak and Longino (1987) outline a possible sequence of three moves by older people. The first move is often to seek amenities, such as better housing, warmer weather, or continuation of long-term friendships. The second "dependence" move may occur after an older person develops a chronic illness and requires assistance. This move may bring the older person into closer proximity to their children or close relatives who can provide this assistance. The third move is often from a community setting to an institutional setting, and usually occurs within a geographically limited area.

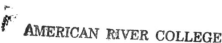 AMERICAN RIVER COLLEGE

101

The classification of internal migration into amenity and dependence moves has validity for the ethnic aged, but all three of these moves do not necessarily occur in all families. Many elderly never make any of these moves. Others make the initial amenity move, but never move again, even if their need for assistance increases dramatically. In other cases, an older person may proceed directly from their first amenity move to a nursing home. The Litwak and Longino classification also neglects the possibility that ethnic aged persons may not be independent decision-makers about their move. Instead, the older Cuban or Haitian man or woman may move from Florida with their children. This move may result from the children's decision to move to another area because of better job opportunities. The likelihood of the older family member joining the children in this move is increased if the older person has health and mental health needs that require extensive assistance.

Migration to Urban Areas

In addition to these types of moves, many older persons have been part of the national trend that has seen a shift in population concentrations from rural small towns to urban metropolitan areas. This shift has occurred among Native Americans, who have relocated from reservations to cities such as Los Angeles. It has also occurred among older African Americans, who, during the period of the First or Second World War, moved from the rural South to northern cities, for jobs in the automobile and steel industries. Recent immigrants arriving from small villages in Central and South America, Africa, or Southeast Asia also face the necessity of adapting to urban life.

Many writers have viewed the position of the older person as downgraded in urbanized society. Cowgill (1988) is the foremost writer on the effects of changes in industrialized urbanized society on the aging. His description indicates a basically negative outcome for the older person.

Urbanization has mixed blessings for older people, who are often left behind as younger people move to large cities to seek work. As already noted, until recently, modern cities have not examined how to make the urban environment convenient, comfortable, and safe for older people. Housing in cities rarely accommodates extended families, because the housing units are frequently too small, expensive, and poorly arranged for comfortable intergenerational living. The pace of life is too hectic, the traffic flows too heavy, the hazards too demanding of quick reflexes, and the risks of criminal victimization too great. Such an environment limits the participation of older people in community affairs, and drives some into virtual self-imprisonment.

In the urban environment, the ethnic aged face major hurdles to maintenance of an independent, satisfying lifestyle. Past practices that have their origin in the ethnic culture may not be adequate to enable the ethnic aged to overcome these hurdles. In rural communities, ethnic families lived together. Some of the norms regarding generational roles may have arisen as efforts to avoid conflict in environments in which individuals lived in close proximity. Even if desired, these close living environments cannot be duplicated in many urban communities. Large families from Southeast Asia cannot live in the same communal and intergenerational arrangements that were typical in their home villages. The cost of housing often makes it impossible for multigenerational families to reside together. Innovative approaches, such as building separate apartments for an older relative onto an existing house, have encountered restrictions based on zoning ordinances, which only allow one-family units in a particular community.

Intergenerational living arrangements may help the older person carry out their daily activities, but this does not guarantee that they will be able to reciprocate the assistance they receive and assist their adult children. The complexity of modern society also makes it difficult for the older person to provide advice to children about taxation, cars, housing, and a myriad of daily issues, particularly if the older person has limited ability in English, as well as limited education. As government programs become more complex, children may be called upon to provide the older person with assistance in understanding and applying for these benefits.

Cowgill emphasizes the heavy traffic flows of urban society as limiting the physical mobility of the aged. As hard as it may be for Americans to imagine, some older immigrants come from cultures where cars are not readily available, and only a small number of people drive. The older ethnic person with limited English fluency may not be able to pass a written test and obtain a driver's license. There are also many older drivers whose reflexes and vision are impaired and should not be driving. The fact that they continue to drive, even with impairments, indicates the dependence of American society on the automobile. Limited physical mobility makes maintaining their social network difficult for many older persons. The telephone enables them to have contact with friends in the community, but face-to-face interaction becomes difficult, if the person cannot drive or does not live in a city with adequate public transportation.

SOCIAL SUPPORT AND THE ELDERLY

The social networks of older persons who cannot drive, or who have limited physical mobility, can quickly become based entirely on family members or friends who live nearby. An older person may have difficulty incorporating new individuals into their social network, if they do not speak English or live in an ethnic enclave.

Social support is necessary at all ages, in order to carry out important tasks. Accomplishing these tasks requires not only the individual's efforts, but also the assistance of other persons in the individual's social network. That network has many functions: It can provide instrumental assistance (task-related assistance) and affective assistance (emotional assistance).

The people who provide these two types of assistance may be the same or different. Some may be persons with whom the older person has regular contact; others may be individuals who the older person has contact with on an occasional basis. Persons with whom the older individual has daily contact may develop into relationships that can be characterized as "strong ties." These are probably not extensive in number, since they are relationships characterized by emotional bonds between individuals. Maintaining these emotional bonds requires an effort on the part of an individual, and this effort limits the number of these relationships. Having strong ties and emotional bonds is crucial in times of crisis, but weak ties have also been shown to be important (Granovetter, 1973). These less emotional relationships may involve people who can be characterized as "acquaintances," but who may provide important information. This information may include leads on new jobs or information about programs of assistance.

The *convoy model* provides a valuable approach to examining the social support networks of older individuals. In the convoy model developed by Kahn and Antonucci (1980), individuals are viewed as having a set of people who provide support at all stages of the life cycle and to whom the person also provides support. The degree to which reciprocity is expected in the giving and receiving of social support may vary according to the ages of the individuals in the social support network. Gouldner (1960) argued that reciprocity is a basic mechanism of society, and that the violation of norms of reciprocity endangers interrelationships. Examined from an exchange theory perspective, the question becomes, What is expected and what is actually being exchanged in the relationships of an older person?

These expectations and actual exchanges may also vary according to ethnic culture. In all cultures, a vital element in the convoy model is the family, which is only one major social institution in society. Others commonly cited include religious organizations and schools. This chapter examines the family and religious organizations and their roles in meeting the needs of the older person, through social support. The questions that need to be explored are:

- What forms of social support do older persons in different ethnic groups desire from their family?
- What factors enable the family to provide needed social support to the older person?
- What factors hamper the ability of the family to provide needed social support to the older person?
- How are these factors related to the ethnic culture and the structure of American society?
- What changes in the ability of the family to provide social support can be projected for the future?
- What roles do religious organizations have in providing social support to the older person?
- What is the relationship of religious organizations as social support mechanisms to the ethnic culture of the older person?
- What changes can be projected in the efforts of religious organizations to provide social support for ethnic elderly?

FAMILY AND THE ETHNIC ELDERLY

For many ethnic aged, the family is the crucial element in meeting the challenges of aging in American society. The family remains the first line of defense against the onset of serious problems among older people. As would be expected, not all members of a family share equally in assisting the older person. Cantor (1979) postulates a pattern of hierarchical compensation as operational in family caregiving patterns. Under this system, the spouse of an older person is initially called upon to provide help if needed. If a spouse is unable or unwilling, adult children become the mainstays of assistance to the older person. As Matthews (1995) and Brotman (2002) have noted, sons and daughters often provide different forms of assistance to their older parents. If sons and daughters are not available, siblings and other relatives move into the position of caregivers. The validity of this hierarchical compensation model, for family assistance among African American, Latino, and Native American families, has been questioned.

There may be differences in family configuration and norms about family assistance that affect the provision of assistance. In addition, the ability of individual family members to provide needed assistance is affected by the proximity of the older person to the family, attitudes of the prospective helper and the older person, and the expertise of the helper. Since ethnic cultures differ on all of these dimensions, we can also expect the configuration of family assistance to the older person to differ among various cultures.

Living Patterns and Social Contact

A strong orientation to the family is characteristic of many ethnic cultures, but there are differences in the amount of contact that occurs between children and parents, and among relatives in general. Italians live in closer proximity to family members than is often found among other Euro-American populations (Cohler & Lieberman, 1979; Johnson, 1985). In Rhode Island, Merrill and Dill (1989) found that Italians, as well as French Canadians, were more likely to have mothers or mothers-in-law living with them than were Irish or Portuguese families. In New Jersey, Johnson (1978) found older Italians more integrated into activities of the family than is common among other ethnic groups. The older Italians also had more frequent contact with their children. Widowed parents were less likely to live alone than widowed parents in other groups. Older people have often been assumed to live with other family members because they do not have the financial resources to afford their own residence. Among Italians, residential patterns could not be explained in these terms.

Examining overall differences in living arrangements of White and non-White older women, Choi (1991) found that the number of children, and duration of widowhood, were the most important factors in determining whether older women will live alone. The non-White sample in Choi's research was predominantly Black women (87%). African American elderly are more likely than Whites to live in extended families, less likely to live alone, and more likely to reside with children and grandchildren (Chatters & Taylor, 1990).

Latino families still tend to live in close proximity to their older relatives. In contrast to other groups, nearly one third of the Latino elderly interviewed by the Commonwealth Fund Commission lived with a child—a percentage twice as great as other groups (Commonwealth Fund Commission on Elderly People Living Alone, 1989). This finding is buttressed by Garcia's (1991) study of 48 residential units on a block in a Latino neighborhood. Garcia found that only 5 of the 40 families had grandparents living with them, but that none of the grandparents lived alone. Instead, these older individuals lived with other adult children. Because of the high fertility rate among Mexican Americans, the probability of adult children having an older person living with them is less than among groups with smaller numbers of children. In contrast to the residential patterns, all of the families qualified as "extended," based on a criterion of interaction and exchange of resources with other kin.

Among Native Americans, family living patterns differ according to reservation or urban residence. Half of the urban Native American population over age 75 lives with other family members, and one third live alone (Kramer, Polisar, & Hyde, 1990). Overall, Native American and Alaskan Native older persons are four times as likely to live with other family members than Whites (Polacca, 2001). As Cuellar's (1990) review indicates, rural-based Native Americans are more likely to live with other family members than Native Americans in cities. Among the Ponca Indians of Oklahoma, living in a rural but nonreservation area, grandchildren were present in 32% of the households of the older respondents. All of the widowed older Native Americans were living in a household with others. This was not true of older Native Americans who had never married, or who were divorced or separated. Among this group, 33% were living alone (John, 1991).

The proportion of Asians living in extended family arrangements has been higher than the national average (Kii, 1984). In some locales, however, the majority of Asian elderly appear to live alone. This pattern is, in part, a reflection of the suburbanization of younger Asian American families. As Kii (1984) notes,

> Many elderly Chinese prefer living in ethnic communities, where they are familiar with the social world and can interact with people using Chinese tongues, to living with their children and the children's families, many of whom have moved to the suburbs or the outskirts of ethnic communities. (p. 210)

Chan (1983) found these factors very important among Chinese elderly in Montreal. Some older Chinese sacrificed the material comforts available through living with their children for the lower housing standards of Chinatown. Conflicts with children and a lack of respect were cited by some of Chan's respondents as factors in the decision to live in Chinatown. The older Chinese also found it difficult to meet Chinese friends in the car-dependent suburbs, or to get to Chinatown for shopping. In Chinatown, older persons were able to easily visit with other Chinese elderly, and to live in close proximity to religious organizations as well as community and social services.

A shift to living alone is also apparent among Korean elderly. Although the elderly would be expected to live with their children in Korea, this pattern is less common in the United States (Min, 1998). Older individuals may live initially with their children, but then establish separate residences as they become acclimated to the United States. This pattern has been found among the Korean immigrant elderly (Kim & Kim, 2001). Socioeconomic factors are important in the decision and the ability of older Koreans to live independently. College-educated Koreans and those with higher incomes were more likely to live alone (Yoo & Sung, 1997).

A comparative analysis of 1990 census data attempted to compare the multigenerational living arrangements of older immigrants across many ethnic groups. Latinos and Asians were more likely to live with family members than were other groups. This pattern was not consistent, however, within each of these groups. Cuban and Japanese older immigrants were less likely to live with younger family members than were other Latinos or Asians. Acculturation to American norms tended to decrease the likelihood of multigenerational households. Entering the United States after the age of 60, and having limited resources and significant needs, increased the likelihood of the older person living with other family members. If older immigrants and their families continue to have problems obtaining health and social welfare benefits and have limited resources of their own, the numbers of older immigrants living with children could continue to increase during the next decades (Wilmoth, 2001).

FAMILY ASSISTANCE PATTERNS

Filial responsibility (the responsibility of children to their parents) is an important norm among many ethnic groups. In part, filial responsibility accounts for the assistance that many families provide older parents. A study of Italian families in Australia revealed major adherence to norms of filial responsibility (McCallum & Gelfand, 1990). The most impressive indicator of filial responsibility was the caregiving that some women had provided their parents for over 20 years. The hardships that the parents endured as a result of migration from Italy to Australia encouraged intensive caregiving on the part of the children. For the women caregivers, there was also no perceived alternative, since nursing homes were not considered acceptable care arrangements.

Positive attitudes toward nursing homes were found among Jewish women caregivers in Australia. As one woman said: "I think that the Jewish nursing home is absolutely marvelous and that my mother is very happy there actually. She says 'I'm not lonely anymore' and I was the one who cried when she went in for four weeks" (McCallum & Gelfand, 1990, p. 23). As a relatively affluent population within Australia, Jews have both positive attitudes toward both formal services and the ability to pay for them.

Aging, Migration, and Ethnicity

Many of the ethnic aged who undertake moves in search of amenities have substantial incomes and pensions. In other cases, ethnic aged with limited incomes have moved from high-cost areas to areas such as the Ozarks, where overall living costs are lower. As these ethnic aged migrate to new areas, a substantial segment of elderly remain behind in the old neighborhoods. In many cases, their children have left the neighborhood in search of better housing or new job opportunities. These migration patterns result in communities with a high percentage of older, lower-income adults.

As older individuals move to new areas, their ethnic background may provide a means of establishing a sense of commonality in a their new community. The presence of a substantial number of individuals from the same ethnic background may also be a factor in the choice of relocation site by older individuals. Stoller (1987) points to the use of ethnic identity as a means of structuring a sense of community among Finns who resettled in Florida. Older individuals who migrate to another area may leave families and friends behind. Because of these losses in their social support network, these migrants could be expected to become more involved in a social support system that included non-kin, such as friends, neighbors, and acquaintances. This pattern was not found among the Finns who relocated to Florida (Stoller, 1998), and may indicate that social support networks can only be built up over a lengthy period of time.

Whatever its size, this Finnish community will not reproduce the ethnic community of new immigrants in its poverty, use of mother tongue, or ethnic institutions. Communities based on the migration of older people will also not reproduce the immigrant ethnic communities with their large numbers of children.

The dispersal of Jews, Finns, and other middle-class White ethnic elderly throughout the country, while their children live at considerable distances, creates new service-delivery problems. In some instances, other relatives are available to help the older person, but this is more the exception than the rule. In most cases, substantial geographic distances between children and older parents places the burden for the provision of care squarely on the shoulders of formal programs and services. This dependence is particularly strong when the older person and their family have not moved within closer geographic proximity in order to meet dependence needs. The ability of the family to dispense the assistance needed by the ethnic aged is clarified by an examination of the situation among specific groups.

AFRICAN AMERICAN FAMILIES AND ASSISTANCE

In contrast to White families, the trend toward greater reliance on formal services is less clear among African Americans. The African American family has always been seen as a buffer for meeting the demands of a White-dominated society. Many researchers argue that slavery destroyed the African American family, because marriages among slaves were not recognized. Other historians believe that the forms of the family brought to the United States from different parts of Africa were distinct from the White European family. Under slavery, only a concerted effort by family members allowed individuals to survive: "The individual was not socialized—nor afforded the opportunity—by his underground community and the mainstream society to 'make it' on his own" (Dilworth-Anderson, 1992, p. 30). The extended networks of African American families also included nonblood-relative individuals, or "fictive kin." In one national survey, 45% of African Americans had fictive kin with whom they maintained active relationships (Chatters, Taylor, & Jayakody, 1994). Among individuals over the age of 85, Johnson (1999) found strong involvement of African Americans with extended families, as well as strong utilization of fictive kin for social support. The use of phrases such as "They are my family," "They are like my family," and "She is a daughter, because she helps me" (p. S372), are all indicators of these fictive kin relationships.

Support Patterns

Despite generally lower income levels, the African American family provides the major share of assistance to the older person. African American families accept their role as caregivers for older members, and may feel it to be a source of emotional rewards (White, Townsend, & Stephens, 2000). Data from the NSBA indicates that older Blacks adhere to the principle of substitution in their choice of helpers (Chatters, Taylor, & Jackson, 1986). Daughters were most often selected as helpers, with sons and spouses the next most frequent choices. Among married individuals, spouses were the most frequently chosen helpers. Divorced older Blacks were more likely to choose a sister as a helper than were separated or widowed respondents, who were more likely to choose a friend as a helper. These choices were consistent, regardless of the age, sex, or socioeconomic status of the respondents. Men, however, were less likely than women to choose daughters as helpers. A study of Whites and African Americans between the ages of 20 and 93 found that there were no significant differences in size of the two groups' social networks. African Americans, however, had more women in their closest relationships (their inner circle), and knew these women for a longer period of time than was true among Whites in the research (Ajrouch, Langfahl, & Antonucci, 2001).

Family caregiving for older African Americans has been categorized as primary, secondary, and tertiary (Dilworth-Anderson, Williams, & Cooper, 1999). Primary caregivers have the highest level of responsibility for a family member and carry out their functions alone or with assistance. Secondary caregivers may perform similar tasks, but do not have the same level of responsibility as the primary caregiver. Tertiary caregivers work with the primary caregiver to provide assistance, but do not bear responsibility for decision-making regarding care. Adult children were the predominant primary, as well as secondary, caregivers, but paid helpers were also significant as secondary caregivers. Tertiary caregivers include adult children, grandchildren, friends, other kin, and paid help.

Family Stresses and Resources

Despite the strong connection of the older African American person to the family, efforts to meet the needs of both younger and older generations are stressful. As Allen (cited in Gibson, 1986a) comments:

There is only so much that one has in the way of economic, emotional and social responses to assist a larger family system that is beset by some of the ravages of being black in this society. And at the same time that you are trying to provide that assistance, you have to deal with your own life and reality. (p. 14)

The contacts among generations established by the African American family, and the intergenerational supports among family members, can be viewed as positive. Whether these supports are adequate is unclear. Examining the NSBA, Gibson (1988) raised questions about the adequacy of the support that can be provided by, and to, the older African American family member. Among older individuals particularly in need are those she terms the "unretired-retired" (1988, p. 304). These older African American men and women are not employed, have discontinuous work histories, and, in many cases, view themselves as disabled.

Fertility rates nationwide declined during the 1980s, but the number of Black children is decreasing more slowly than the number of White children. Black elderly, therefore, have larger potential pools of support from children than do Whites. But in order to provide the needed support, these children require adequate socioeconomic resources, and at this point in time, their resources may not be sufficient. The increase in single mothers living in poverty means less capability on the part of African American adult children to address the needs of their older parents. This lessened capability may account for national data that indicate lower levels of intergenerational assistance among African Americans than among Mexican Americans or Whites. To compensate, the extended kin network will be required to play an increasing role in the provision of assistance for the older African American (Dilworth-Anderson, 1992). As McAdoo (1998) has noted, declines in marriage rates among African Americans, and economic problems, are major threats to the resiliency of the traditional Black extended family. The role of fictive kin in compensating for these changes needs to be explored (Johnson, 1999).

African Americans have been able to draw upon a more diverse group of helpers for assistance, and to interchange these helpers as needed, than have Whites or Latino (Gibson & Jackson, 1987; Hatch, 1990). A restudy of older persons in New York City indicates that this situation is as true in the 1990s as it was in the 1970s (Cantor, 1992, 1995). Whether these additional helpers, many of whom are extended family members, are able to relieve pressures on the family, arising from the needs of the older person, children, and grandchildren, remains to be determined. MaloneBeach and Cook (2001) raise the interesting question of whether extensive social support from African American women, in the form of caregiving, is part of the legacy of African Americans. In this sense, women caregiving for older parents is only part of a tradition of caregiving, which at different times may include siblings, their own children, nieces and nephews, grandparents, and parents. How extensive this legacy is, and whether it will continue among African Americans, can only be studied over time.

LATINO FAMILIES AND ASSISTANCE

Familismo, which can be defined as "strong feeling of reciprocity and solidarity among family members" (Ayalon, Lopez, Huyck, & Yoder, 2001, p. 2) is a basic value among Latino ethnic groups. As is true of the African American family, the Latino family in the United States is a social system faced with needs at both ends of the age spectrum. Older people require assistance to meet functional needs as well as the psychological process of aging. Young children require nurturing, educational opportunities, and health care. Many Latino parents do not possess the resources necessary to meet all of these demands.

Latino Family Configurations

The use of a larger network of individuals helps to compensate for the lack of socioeconomic resources among many Latino families. In many Western societies, the concept of family has tended to be confined to blood relatives but in Latino cultures, the concept of family can include a wider segment of the population. As Becerra (1998) describe its evolution:

> For the traditional Mexican, the word family meant an extended multigenerational group of persons, with specific social roles ascribed to members of each age group. By dividing functions and responsibilities among different generations of family members, the family was able to perform all the economic and social support chores necessary for survival in the relatively spartan life circumstances of the rural Mexican environment. Mutual support, sustenance and interaction during both work and leisure hours dominated the lives of persons in these traditional Mexican families. (p. 158)

Examining the Puerto Rican family, Sanchez-Ayendez (1998) questions the idea of a family that can be termed *traditional*. Socioeconomic conditions have affected the nature of the Puerto Rican family over time. As is common in many Latino cultures, the fictive kin network includes individuals who are not related by blood and who are brought into the family through rituals that make them coparents (*compadrazgo*). Valle (1983) has shown how the compadre is used to provide assistance to elderly individuals.

The level of assistance available from family varies for older persons in rural and urban communities. In the urban barrio, the older Latino may have a substantial number of friends and nonrelatives who provide assistance. In rural areas, the family may be even more important as a source of assistance. A study of assistance patterns among Latinos in rural Colorado indicated extensive linkages between Mexican elderly and their family (Magilvy, Congdon, Martinez, Davis, & Averill, 2000).

> Among the older Latino participants in the study, nearly every one had a spouse, adult child, sibling niece or nephew, or grandchild living nearby. Relatives or friends often dropped in for a visit during our home, hospital or nursing home visits. Close family members had daily contact with one another via telephone or in person, and elders whose adult children lived outside the community maintained contact by regular telephone calls and frequent visits. (p. 178)

This high level of contact may, in part, explain why decision-making about appropriate care for an older person has been found to be made by the family unit, rather than only by the individual caregiver (Ayalon et al., 2001).

Changes in Family Assistance Patterns

As is true of all ethnic groups, family patterns may change in response to changes in the society. In the Cuban American family, the need to recover economically from the losses encountered when leaving Cuba, and the materialism of American culture, have been seen as eroding the time Cubans are willing to spend interacting with their family. In addition, many younger Cubans have moved away from their families in order to pursue education and job opportunities (Suarez, 1998). These changes may be less evident among Puerto Rican families, because they have easy access to Puerto Rico and do not have any concerns about obtaining citizenship status (Sanchez-Ayendez, 1998).

In New York City, assistance for Puerto Rican elderly who patronized a hospital-based geriatric clinic was provided predominantly by kin (Cairo, Libhber, & Felton, 1992). Among Mexican Americans in the San Antonio area (Talamantes, Espino, Cornell, Lichtenstein, & Hazuda, 1992), a spouse, children, and other blood relatives, rather than extended or nonblood-related individuals, predominated as caregivers. Nationally, data from the National Survey of Families and Households does not indicate higher levels of support among Mexican American children and parents than is found among other groups (Eggebeen, 1992). An extensive review of studies of caregiving among various ethnic groups has also noted conflicting results. In some of the research reviewed, few Latino respondents relied on non-kin for assistance with long-term impairments, but, in others, almost one third of the respondents cared for themselves after hospitalization (Aranda & Knight, 1997).

Latino elders do not appear to expect family members to meet their needs without assistance from formal programs. In fact, some past research indicated that Latino elders have higher expectations of assistance from the government than other groups (Crouch, 1982). These expectations are not necessarily related to income levels of the older person (Cox & Gelfand, 1987). Expectations differ, however, according to whether the older Latinos were born in or outside the United States. The expectation of government support may account for Baker's (1984) finding that Mexican American elderly, receiving home care in Arizona, also received less assistance from spouses, relatives, and friends than did Anglo clients.

In San Antonio, lower- and middle-class Mexican Americans were less likely than those of their more affluent peers to "perceive that they had an available caregiver" (Talamantes, Cornell, Espino, Lichtenstein, & Hazuda, 1996, p. 96). Among the 309 Mexican Americans in the research, 30% felt that they would not have a caregiver available if they became seriously ill. The researchers suggest that these older Mexican Americans may be reluctant to call upon family members for assistance, since they could not provide the reciprocal support that is part of the cultural tradition.

Even if the values of the extended family are adhered to, recent Latino immigrants may have lost touch with many of the family's members. Immigration forces the breakup of many families. If a chain migration, typical of most immigrant groups, is followed, a man or woman may come alone to the United States to seek work. An undocumented worker may have left the family behind because of the difficulties involved in crossing the border. At a later date, when settled, the immigrant may send for other members of the family. This process is abetted if immigrants are able to obtain permanent resident, then U.S. citizenship status, which allows them to bring immediate family members (parents, spouses, children) into the country under family reunification preferences. If the extended family is not recreated in the United States, the Latino immigrants may have less support available when the older family member needs assistance. Among recent immigrants able to bring their family intact into the country, interaction patterns may be extensive, unless family members begin to migrate to other communities. A New York City study of African American, Latino, and White elderly found Latinos to be the most family-centered of the three groups, to have more children living nearby, and to have a larger network of siblings (Cantor, 1992, 1995). The recent immigration of many of the Latino families may partially explain these strong family relationships.

NATIVE AMERICAN FAMILIES AND ASSISTANCE

Reservation and Nonreservation Families

Traditionally, the assumption has been that Native American families are primarily family-dependent support networks. The family network, however, cannot be subsumed under a European-based model of kinship, but may include a larger framework built around a village model. Red Horse, Lewis, Feit, and Decker (1978) and Williams (1980) argue that the household is an inappropriate measure of family extension among Native Americans. Several households may be included within the family network (Red Horse et al., 1978). Little is known regarding the extent to which other forms of social support networks are developing, as changes occur on reservations and among Native American families living in urban and rural areas. Many American Indians have moved to urban areas, because of job opportunities (Ablon, 1965). The model of the large intergenerational Native American household has been labeled a stereotype inapplicable in urban Native American communities (Weibel-Orlando & Kramer, 1989). As a result of changes in these social networks, there may be more or less formal care provided by the network. The specific individuals who provide this assistance may also change.

Native Americans living in urban areas may be more isolated from their family members living on the reservation. Some of these differences were evident in a study done in Oregon and Washington (Manson, 1984). Asked about their most important persons, 75% of the older Native Americans interviewed in the city, versus 89% of those interviewed on the reservation, stressed family as their important persons.

On a number of problems, urban Native American elderly reported less available social resources.

John (1998) has, however, questioned the traditional view of the cohesive extended Native American family. In his view, the current literature does not adequately probe the family changes that are occurring as a result of a growing number of urbanized Native Americans and underestimates the needs of Native American elderly:

> The idea that the mere existence of an extended family is sufficient to meet the needs of elders places a number of them at risk, since the extended family is not a universal feature in the lives of either rural or urban American Indians. (p. 409)

Native Americans in urban areas rely more on the formal service-delivery system than do their reservation peers. Although the demands on the family are greater on reservations than in urban areas, the family is a crucial provider of assistance in both environments. Even with the commitment of the family, assistance to older persons may not be optimal. Among Oneidas in Wisconsin, Kapke found strong intergenerational links, but a failure on the part of extended families to follow through or communicate when an older person needed assistance (Kapke, 1988).

As is true among Latinos, Native Americans may view the family from a perspective that goes beyond blood-related individuals. In a small study of Native American aged in Montana, respondents viewed family as including kin and non-kin, as well as individuals in the community with whom they had relationships (Wallace & Bergeman, 2001).

ASIAN FAMILIES AND ASSISTANCE

Traditional values in many Asian cultures stress family allegiance as a core value. As Sue (1989) describes Asian cultural values:

> The inculcation of guilt and shame are the principal techniques used to control the behavior of family members. Parents emphasize their children's obligation to the family. If a child acts independently (contrary to the wishes of his parents) he is told he is selfish and inconsiderate and that he is not showing gratitude for all his parents have done for them. The behavior of individual members of an Asian family is expected to reflect credit on the whole family. (p. 104)

In traditional Asian cultures, not providing assistance to parents would reflect negatively on the whole family.

Indications are that these traditional norms are beginning to attenuate, in both the United States and Asia. The factors producing this change are not greatly different on both continents and include movement of children and family away from each other, larger numbers of women in the work force unable to provide care to their parents, and unavailability of housing units that allow for intergenerational living. In the United States, Yu (cited in Morioka-Douglas & Yeo, 1990) found that fewer than half of the midwestern Chinese American respondents expressed strong adherence to filial beliefs. Among the women over age 36, more indicated that they were assisting parents than expressed belief in norms of filial piety.

A study of older Vietnamese in Texas (Die & Seelbach, 1988) found that most of the older Texan Vietnamese respondents lived with their children, a living pattern that naturally promotes extensive intergenerational contact. These older Vietnamese had migrated with their children, and 62% of the sample of 60 persons had 5 or more children in the United States. Not all of these children lived in close proximity to the older parents.

These older parents adhered to traditional norms about the role of children: Over 90% believed that older persons should live with children when unable to take care of themselves or if they did not want to live alone. A similar unanimity was found in the belief that one major function of children was to provide care for aging parents. Whether these attitudes will persist among succeeding generations of Vietnamese is unclear. Some indications of change in attitudes toward aging among Asians are found in a study of Cambodian elderly. As Becker and Beyene (1999) report, many of the older Cambodians interviewed were upset with what they regarded as changes in attitudes among the children, but, particularly, their grandchildren. The older Cambodians did not feel they received the respect that should be accorded the elderly. An inability on the part of the grandchildren to speak Cambodian also made it impossible for the monolingual grandparents to communicate with them, except through gestures.

Structural Changes and Norms

Norms about assistance may remain stable, but structural conditions, such as the work situation of women, may make full compliance with these norms difficult. Alternatively, the norms of filial obligation may decline among younger generations, but families may continue to provide the bulk of care to parents, because of problems in obtaining needed formal services. This pattern is consistent with Rosenthal's (1986) assertion that variations in norms of filial responsibility do not necessarily correspond with differences in filial support. Whatever the reasons for this disparity, older parents may still be distressed when children are unable to provide the support and assistance they need.

Older Asians provide an example of the gaps between the needs and assistance received by the ethnic aged. Yeo (1992) has provided a good summary of these gaps. As she noted, many older Asians who have followed their children to the United States suffer from multiple isolation patterns. These include isolation from:

- family in the home country
- community and other traditional family supports
- the new community in the United States (unless they are living in a predominantly Asian community)
- children they followed to the United States (since these children may be at work while the older person remains at home to provide child care)
- acculturated grandchildren whose values are different and who may not even speak the mother tongue

THE OLDER PERSON AS PROVIDER

A focus on the assistance provided to the older person omits the assistance that these individuals, in all ethnic and racial groups, provide to their children. In some cases, the older person may become the de facto parent of the children, as young parents find themselves unable to cope with the demands of childrearing or become victims of drug abuse or other destructive habits. In many cases, older people may find that their children have moved back home with them.

Older African Americans raising grandchildren has become increasingly more common in the United States, increasing from 3.2% in 1970 to 5.4% of all households in 1994 (Lugaila, 1998). A national survey of over 3,000 grandparents found that African Americans were twice as likely as other groups to take on full parenting roles (Fuller-Thomson, Minkler, & Driver, 1997).

The care that older African Americans provide for grandchildren is an extension of the historically important role of grandparents in the African American family. Although there are clearly emotional rewards for surrogate parenting, it takes its toll on the older person, most of whom are women. Some grandparents have given up jobs to take on the parenting role. Others find the physical demands of coping with a young child difficult; all find that the day-to-day demands of parenting result in a loss of free time and opportunities to interact with friends and family (Burton & Devries, 1992).

There may be differences in the impact of parenting between "living-with" grandparents and "custodial grandparents" (Jendrek, 1993). Living-with grandparents and custodial grandparents may have the same roles, but custodial grandparents have legal custody of their grandchildren. The demands on grandparents were found to be more significant among custodial grandparents, and ranged from weakened relationships with family and friends, to less privacy, less time for leisure activities, and less money. Pruchno (1999) has documented the toll among working women. The negative impacts included having to stay home or being late for work. For African American custodial grandparents, the negative impacts were heightened, because they were more likely to be divorced or widowed than their White counterparts.

Financial support for children has been more feasible for economically successful groups such as Italians and Jews, but is also common among all ethnic groups. Among Native Americans, coresidence of the elderly with grandchildren is common. As is often the case with Latinos, whose home the older person is living in is not always evident.

RELIGION AND THE ETHNIC AGED

The strength of social institutions, such as religious organizations and the family, is often related to an ethnic group's history. Expectations about assistance from the religious organization may also vary among ethnic groups. These expectations are based on religious attitudes and beliefs, as well as on traditional patterns of service delivery from the religious organization. Jewish, Catholic, and African American communal organizations have taken on responsibility for providing services to the aged, but the Mormon Church places responsibility for assistance to older people on the family (Campbell & Campbell, 1998; Gelfand & Olsen, 1979). This emphasis on the family is consistent with Mormon religious beliefs, which stress the primacy of the family in all aspects of life. The Amish religion also emphasizes the responsibility of the family to care for the infirm or poor older person, but with assistance from the church. The Amish elderly retire at home and are cared for by children. If the burden of care is great, families may take turns assisting the older person, since the use of residential institutions is not allowed.

Additional funds required by a widow(er) are provided through the Amish community (Kraybill, 1989).

African American Aged and Religion

As a major community institution, religious organizations are probably most important among African Americans. As Foner (1988) notes, churches began to develop among freedmen soon after the end of the Civil War. Churches represented the only community institution not controlled by Whites. In many communities, churches have remained independent of any political structure.

Religious involvement is high among African Americans of all ages. The NSBA found that 40% of the respondents attended church weekly, and that 70% attended services at least a few times a month. Two thirds of Black adults were also church members, and viewed the church as a vital element in economic, social, and political progress for the African American community (Chatters & Taylor, 1989). Religious involvement, in both organized and nonorganized forms, among African Americans, increased with age. The highest levels of involvement were, in fact, among the oldest age cohorts in the national survey:

> The conventional wisdom that individuals become more concerned with religious matters as they grow older may be a valid portrayal of the experience of Black Americans, and it is suggested that age change is an important component of age differences in religious involvement. (Chatters & Taylor, 1989, p. S158)

A further analysis of the NSBA (Krause & Tran, 1989) supports the hypothesis that religious involvement of older African Americans reduces the effects of stressors such as financial problems, difficulties with health, and racial problems. Whether religious involvement has the same effect, over a wide range of stressors, remains untested. An analysis of national data suggests that involvement in church social events helps older African American women maintain an informal support network that extends beyond family members (Hatch, 1990). Hatch's research confirms earlier studies in Alabama (Ortega, Crutchfield, & Rushing, 1983), which also found that older African American women are more active in religious organizations than their male counterparts.

It would be a mistake, however, to stress only the organizational influence of religious organizations on the lives of African American elderly. Prayer serves as a coping mechanism (Husaini, Castor, Linn,

Whitten-Stovall, & Neser, 1988) for older Blacks and older Whites (Husaini, Moore, & Cain, 1991; Koenig, George, & Sigler, 1988). The use of prayer as help-seeking behavior is stronger among Black and White older women than it is among men. Prayer may also partly account for the lower rate of suicide among Black, compared to White, elderly (Gibson, 1986b), and church attendance has been found to be related to a reduced risk of mortality among older African Americans (Bryant & Rakowski, 1992). As these authors note, this effect probably reflects the role of the church as a provider of informal and formal support for its members.

Latino and Native American Aged and Religion

Among Latinos and Native Americans, religion is not a pure concept, since orthodox religious practices have often been combined with indigenous beliefs. For example, Catholicism is the dominant organized religion among Latinos, and its religious practices certainly fit this pattern. Among Puerto Ricans, Catholicism is mixed with spiritualism (Sanchez-Ayendez, 1998). Spiritualism also plays an important role among Mexicans. In recent years, Protestant evangelicals have been active among Latino groups. A National Hispanic Council on Aging study of Latino elderly, in four American locations, indicates that 18% of the sample are Protestants (Gallego, 1988).

A variety of Protestant and Catholic groups have a long history of missionary and evangelical efforts among Native Americans. The Mormon Church has been particularly active on Indian reservations. Church-operated boarding schools are a major element in Native American history, but the involvement of religious institutions in service delivery varies by denomination. Besides specific denominations, there are a variety of religious beliefs among Native Americans that focus on the need to maintain harmony between humans, nature, and the supernatural.

Asian Aged and Religion

The importance of religion for Asian elderly is impossible to discuss briefly, because of the extensive number of religions, which include Christianity, Buddhism, Hinduism, and Shintoism. Confucianism, which has a long history in Chinese society, is not a religion, but a strong belief system that lays down norms of behavior and family roles and obligations. In China and some other Asian societies, Confucianism, rather than an organized religious system, has been the guiding principle of the society. Confucianism includes age-graded norms that stress the authority of the elder, respect for the elderly, and the family obligation of children to the older person (Min, 1998).

Religion and Life Satisfaction

The religious involvement of older people can be an important factor in their life satisfaction. In a large sample that included rural and urban older Blacks and Whites, Blacks evidenced a higher degree of life satisfaction. Analysis indicated that this difference was explained by more extensive contact of older African Americans with church friends, even though the older White respondents had a larger number of friends. In the South, religious groups may provide a "pseudo-family," particularly for African American elderly whose children have moved to the North (Ortega et al., 1983). This role for the church was not confirmed by NSBA data (Smith, 1993). The church did, however, provide a base for a larger social support network: 80% of the Black elderly in the sample received support from a best friend or close friend, 60% from church members, and 50% from extended family members (Chatters & Taylor, 1998).

Data regarding the effects of religious involvement on the life satisfaction of older Latinos is not consistent. Among Mexican Americans, religious attendance was a strong predictor of life satisfaction for older women, but not for older men (Levin & Markides, 1988).

The importance of religious involvement for the ethnic aged is not always easy to discern, because membership in a religious organization, attendance at religious services, and the meaning of religion are not always synonymous. In the National Hispanic Council on Aging study of Mexican Americans and Puerto Ricans over the age of 65, half of the sample attended church less often than they did when they were 55 years old. Men attended church less often than women. The major reasons for not attending church were the same for both men and women: lack of transportation and physical problems (Gallego, 1988).

Religious Organizations and Aging Services

Regardless of the extent of the older individual's participation in religious services or activities conducted by religious organizations, they may view the religious organization as a provider of direct services or as an organization legitimizing services. Social welfare agencies affiliated with religious groups, such as Catholic Charities, are significant providers of social and health services in American cities. Even if they do not provide the actual services, religious organizations may provide space for programs operated by local social welfare agencies. In many communities, health and mental health organizations view churches as major sources of outreach to ethnic aged. The emphasis of religiously based services, however, is often not older people, but children and young families. If only 8% of the services provided by African American churches are directed toward older persons, the role of the Black church as a major source of support can be questioned (Dilworth-Anderson, Williams, & Williams, 2001).

For recent immigrant aged, a religious organization may play a unique role in resettlement and acculturation activities. One example is Korean Christian churches, which are predominantly Protestant in background. These churches are important to Koreans not only because of their religious values, but also because they provide the Korean immigrant with a sense of identity: "In addition, they provide a place for meeting people and a sanctuary for obtaining peace of mind and self-improvement" (Kitano, 1988, p. 114).

Regardless of their training, ministers may be called upon to act as a mental health resource by older persons. In Nashville, clergy were more likely than physicians to be called upon by African American elderly (36.9% vs. 30.8%), to respond to problems of worry, nerves, and emotional stress. The use of the clergy as a mental health resource was higher among Black than White elderly (37% vs. 24%) (Husaini et al., 1988).

Starret, Sousa, Decker, Walter, and Keller (n.d.) have found that Latino elderly use religious organizations twice as often as any other sources of assistance. This usage pattern is modified when the ability of the older Latino to obtain assistance is taken into account. Latino elderly who have lived in a community for a substantial length of time tend to make greater use of a physician, rather than clergy, to meet their mental health needs.

Religious Organizations and Public Social Welfare

The involvement of religious organizations in social welfare has strong precedents in American history. As Kutzik (1979) notes, the history of social welfare in the United States has been characterized, for the longest period, by a dependence on sectarian religiously based services. As was true among African American communities, the development of these services was necessary among many ethnic groups, because of the discrimination they faced from the available services. Over the years, these sectarian services have gained in esteem and respect from the public. In contrast, public services in the country have often been viewed as being only a last resort and of poor quality. This attitude was reflected in a survey of Italian men in a suburban Maryland community. In contrast to a sample of inner-city, lower-income Baltimore families, these men expressed some willingness to use formal services for their older parents, when needed. Their primary choices were private and church-related services, because of the higher quality they associated with services under these auspices (Gelfand & Fandetti, 1980).

These choices of private and religious providers may reflect a change in attitudes toward the public social welfare system. During the 1930s, funds from the federal government were crucial in the effort to pull the country out of the depression. In recent years, federal, as well as state and local, government programs have become identified as low-quality efforts for the poor and infirm. This identification is based on limited or invalid evidence, but now appears to be a factor in the negative attitude of many Americans toward increased taxes.

Public and private services for the aged have grown dramatically since the 1960s, when the OAA was passed. Unlike many other services, these efforts have gained a positive reputation among older Americans and service providers in other fields. Whatever their quality, continued support for these services depends on obtaining the involvement of as many older people as require their assistance. Many providers report frustration in their efforts to involve older people or their families in programs and services.

The delay in use of available services, or the failure to use them at all, can have a negative impact on both the older person and their family. Although the provision of care by the family for older persons from various ethnic backgrounds reduces costs for taxpayers, the older person may not receive the quality of care they need from an untrained caregiver. There are also the many personal and social sacrifices that must be made by caregivers to provide intensive care. As family-based care is promoted as the preferable form of caregiving for older persons, innovative approaches to formal care may be overlooked, and needed improvements, in settings such as nursing homes, not undertaken (Strawbridge & Wallhagen, 1992). With its strong emphasis on families and children, Mormon culture may only commit limited resources for family care of the elderly (Campbell, 2001). What is needed is clearly a balance between the informal care that is provided effectively by the older person's social support network and formal care from public and private agencies.

Developing and implementing effective services for the ethnic aged is not a simple task. The next chapter examines the factors that may account for the problems in serving the ethnic aged.

REFERENCES

Ablon, J. (1965). American Indian relocation: Problems of dependency and management in the city. *Phylon, 16,* 362–371.

Ajrouch, K., Langfahl, E., & Antonucci, T. (2001, November). *Close relationships and social networks: A Black-White comparison.* Paper presented at the annual meeting of the Gerontological Society of America, Chicago.

Aranda, M., & Knight, B. (1997). The influence of ethnicity and culture on the caregiver stress and coping process: A sociocultural review and analysis. *The Gerontologist, 37,* 342–354.

Ayalon, L., Lopez, G., Huyck, M., & Yoder, J. (2001, November). *Providing informal care to an elderly family member: The Latino perspective.* Paper presented at the annual meeting of the Gerontological Society, Chicago.

Baker, M. (1984). *Some characteristics of Mexican-American home health care clients in metropolitan Arizona.* Paper presented at the annual meeting of the Gerontological Society of America, San Antonio, TX.

Becerra, R. (1998). The Mexican-American family. In C. Mindel, R. Habenstein, & R. Wright, Jr. (Eds.), *Ethnic families in America: Patterns and variations* (4th ed.) (pp. 153–171). New York: Elsevier.

Becker, G., & Beyene, Y. (1999). Narratives of age and uprootedness among older Cambodian refugees. *Journal of Aging Studies, 13,* 295–314.

Brotman, S. (2002). The primacy of family in elder care discourse: Home care services to older ethnic women in Canada. *Journal of Gerontological Social Work, 38*(3), 19–52.

Burton, L., & Devries, C. (1992). Challenges and rewards: African American grandparents as surrogate parents. *Generations, 17*(3), 51–54.

Bryant, S., & Rakowski, W. (1992). Predictors of mortality among elderly African-Americans. *Research on Aging, 14,* 50–67.

Cairo, L., Libhber, J., & Felton, B. (1992, November). *Roles of kin and nonkin in the social networks of elderly Puerto Ricans.* Paper presented at the annual meeting of the Gerontological Society of America, Washington, DC.

Campbell, B. (2001) Mormon elderly. In L. Olsen (Ed.), *Age through ethnic lenses: Caring for the elderly in a multicultural society* (pp. 123–133). Lanham, MD: Rowman and Littlefield.

Campbell, B., & Campbell, E. (1998). The Mormon family. In C. Mindel, R. Habenstein, & R. Wright, Jr. (Eds.), *Ethnic families in America: Patterns and variations* (4th ed.) (pp. 480–507). New York: Elsevier.

Cantor, M. (1979). Neighbors and friends: An overlooked resource in the informal support system. *Research on Aging, 1,* 434–463.

Cantor, M. (1992, November). *The extent and configuration of informal supports among New York City elderly: Does ethnicity make a difference?* Paper presented at the Gerontological Society of America, Washington, DC.

Cantor, M. (1995). The importance of ethnicity in the social support systems of older New Yorkers: A longitudinal perspective. *Journal of Gerontological Social Work, 22*(3/4), 95–128.

Chan, K. (1983). Coping with aging and managing self-identity: The social world of elderly Chinese women. *Canadian Ethnic Studies, 15,* 36–50.

Chatters, L., & Taylor, R. (1989). Age differences in religious participation among Black adults. *Journals of Gerontology: Social Sciences, 44,* S183–189.

Chatters, L., & Taylor, R. (1990). Social integration. In Z. Harel, E. McKinney, & M. Williams (Eds.), *Black aged: Understanding diversity and service needs* (pp. 63–82). Newbury Park, CA: Sage.

Chatters, L., & Taylor, R. (1998). Religious involvement among African Americans. *African American Research Perspectives.* Retrieved May 20, 2002, from *http://www.rcgd.isr.umich.edu/prba/persp/spring1998*

Chatters, L., Taylor, J., & Jackson, J. (1986). Aged Blacks' choices for an informal helper network. *Journal of Gerontology, 41,* 94–100.

Chatters, L., Taylor, R., & Jayakody, R. (1994). Fictive kinship relationships in black extended families. *Journal of Comparative Family Studies, 25,* 297–312.

Choi, N. (1991). Racial differences in the determinants of living arrangements of widowed and divorced elderly women. *The Gerontologist, 31,* 496–504.

Cohler, B., & Lieberman, M. (1979). Personality change across the second half of life: Findings from a study of Irish, Italian, and Polish-American men and women. In D. Gelfand & A. Kutzik (Eds.), *Ethnicity and aging: Theory, research and policy* (pp. 227–245). New York: Springer Publishing.

Commonwealth Fund Commission on Elderly People Living Alone. (1989). *Poverty and poor health among elderly Hispanic Americans.* Baltimore: Author.

Cowgill, D. (1988). Aging in cross-cultural perspective: Africa and the Americas. In E. Gort (Ed.), *Aging in cross-cultural perspective* (pp. 110–132). New York: Phelps-Stokes Fund.

Cox, C., & Gelfand, D. (1987). Family assistance, exchange and the ethnic elderly. *Journal of Cross-Cultural Gerontology, 2,* 241–256

Crouch, B. (1982). Age and institutional support: Perceptions of older Mexican-Americans. *Journal of Gerontology, 37,* 524–529.

Cuellar, J. (1990). *Aging and health: American Indian/Alaska Native.* Stanford Geriatric Education Center Working Paper Series, Number 6, Ethnogeriatric Reviews. Stanford, CA: Stanford Geriatric Education Center.

Die, A., & Seelbach, W. (1988). Problems, sources of assistance, and knowledge of services among elderly Vietnamese immigrants. *The Gerontologist, 28,* 448–452.

Dilworth-Anderson, P. (1992). Extended networks in Black families. *Generations, 17*(3), 29–32.

Dilworth-Anderson, P., Williams, S., & Cooper, T. (1999). Family caregiving to elderly African Americans: Caregiver types and structures. *Journal of Gerontology: Social Sciences, 54B,* S237–S241.

Dilworth-Anderson, P., Williams, I., & Williams, S. (2001). Urban elderly African Americans. In L. Olsen (Ed.), *Age through ethnic lenses: Caring for the elderly in a multicultural society* (pp. 95–102). Lanham, MD: Rowman and Littlefield.

Eggebeen, D. (1992). From generation unto generation: Parent-child support in aging American families. *Generations, 17*(3), 45–49.

Fuller-Thomson, E., Minkler, M., & Driver, D. (1997). A profile of grandparents raising grandchildren in the United States. *The Gerontologist, 37,* 406–411.

Foner, E. (1988). *Reconstruction: America's unfinished revolution.* New York: Harper and Row.

Gallego, D. (1988). Religiosity as a coping mechanism among Hispanic elderly. In M. Sotomayor & H. Curiel (Eds.), *Hispanic elderly: A cultural signature* (pp. 117–136). Edinburgh, TX: Pan American University Press.

Garcia, C. (1991, November). *The extended family: A closer look at Hispanic multigenerational families.* Paper presented at the annual meeting of the Gerontological Society of America, San Francisco.

Gelfand, D., & Fandetti, D. (1980). Suburban and urban white ethnics: Attitudes towards care of the aged. *The Gerontologist, 20,* 588–594.

Gelfand, D., & Olsen, J. (1979). Aging in the Jewish and the Mormon family. In D. Gelfand & A. Kutzik (Eds.), *Ethnicity and aging: Theory, research and policy* (pp. 206–222). New York: Springer Publishing.

Gibson, R. (1986a). *Blacks in an aging society.* New York: Carnegie Corporation.

Gibson, R. (1986b). Outlook for the Black family. In A. Pifer & L. Bronte (Eds.), *Our aging society.* New York: W. W. Norton.

Gibson, R. (1988). The work, retirement and disability of older Black Americans. In J. Jackson (Ed.), *The Black American elderly: Research on physical and psychosocial health.* New York: Springer Publishing.

Gibson, R., & Jackson, J. (1987). The health, physical functioning, and informal supports of the Black elderly. *The Milbank Quarterly, 65*(Suppl. 2), 421–454.

Gouldner, A. (1960). The norms of reciprocity: A preliminary statement. *American Sociological Review, 25,* 161–178.

Granovetter, M. (1973). The strength of weak ties. *American Sociological Review, 78,* 1360–1380.

Hatch, L. (1990, November). *Informal support patterns of older African American and White women: Examining effects of family, paid work, and religious participation.* Paper presented at the annual meeting of the Gerontological Society of America, Boston.

Husaini, B., Castor, R., Linn, J., Whitten-Stovall, R., & Neser, W. (1988, November). *Psychological well-being and help-seeking behavior among the Black elderly: Gender differences.* Paper presented at the annual meeting of the Gerontological Society of America, San Francisco.

Husaini, B., Moore, S., & Cain, V. (1991). *Psychiatric symptoms and help-seeking behavior among the elderly: Black-White comparisons.* Paper presented at the Historic Black Colleges and Universities Gerontological Association meeting, Norfolk, VA.

Jendrek, M. (1993). Grandparents who parent their grandchildren: Effects on lifestyle. *Journal of Marriage and the Family, 55,* 609–621.

John, R. (1991). *Defining and meeting the needs of Native American elders, Vol. 5: Ponca Tribe of Oklahoma.* Washington, DC: Administration on Aging.

John, R. (1998). The Native American family. In C. Mindel, R. Habenstein, & R. Wright, Jr. (Eds.), *Ethnic families in America: Patterns and variations* (4th ed.) (pp. 382–421). New York: Elsevier.

Johnson, C. (1978). Family support system of elderly Italian-Americans. *Journal of Minority Aging, 3–4,* 34–41.

Johnson, C. (1985). *Growing up and growing old in Italian-American families.* New Brunswick, NJ: Rutgers University Press.

Johnson, C. (1999). Fictive kin among oldest old African Americans in the San Francisco Bay area. *Journal of Gerontology: Social Sciences, 54B,* S368–375.

Kahn, R., & Antonucci, T. (1980). Convoy over the life course: Attachment, roles and social support. In P. Baltes & O. Brim (Eds.), *Life-span development and behavior* (pp. 79–92). New York: Academic Press.

Kapke, K. (1988). *The health status and health service needs of the elderly of the Oneida Indian tribe.* Final report of the Postdoctoral Fellowship Program in Applied Gerontology. Washington, DC: Gerontological Society of America.

Kii, T. (1984). Asians. In E. Palmore (Ed.), *Handbook of the aged in the United States* (pp. 201–208). Westport, CT: Greenwood Press.

Kim, S., & Kim, K. (2001). Intimacy at a distance, Korean American style: Invited Korean elderly and their married children. In L. Olsen (Ed.), *Age through ethnic lenses: Caring for the elderly in a multicultural society* (pp. 45–58). Lanham, MD: Rowman and Littlefield.

Kitano, H. (1988). *Asian Americans: Emerging minorities.* Englewood Cliffs, NJ: Prentice-Hall.

Koenig, H., George, L., & Sigler, I. (1988). The use of religion and other emotion-regulation coping strategies among older adults. *The Gerontologist, 28,* 303–310.

Kramer, B., Polisar, D., & Hyde, J. (1990). *Study of urban American Indian aging:* Final report. City of Industry, CA: The Public Health Foundation.

Krause, N., & Tran, T. (1989). Stress and religious involvement among older Blacks. *Journals of Gerontology: Social Sciences, 44,* S4–13.

Kraybill, D. (1989). *The riddle of Amish culture.* Baltimore: Johns Hopkins University Press.

Kutzik, A. (1979). American social provision for the aged: An historical perspective. In D. Gelfand & A. Kutzik (Eds.), *Ethnicity and aging: Theory, research and policy* (pp. 32–65). New York: Springer Publishing.

Levin, J., & Markides, K. (1988). Religious attendance and psychological well-being in middle-aged and older Mexican Americans. *Sociological Analysis, 49,* 66–72.

Litwak, E., & Longino, C. (1987). Migration patterns among the elderly: A developmental perspective. *The Gerontologist, 27,* 266–272.

Lugaila, T. (1998). *Marital status and living arrangements: March 1997.* Current Population Reports, P 20–154. Washington, DC: U.S. Census Bureau.

Magilvy, J., Congdon, J., Martinez, R., Davis, J., & Averill, D. (2000). Caring for our own: Experiences of rural Hispanic elders. *Journal of Aging Studies, 14,* 171–190.

MaloneBeach, E., & Cook, T. (2001). *African American women: A legacy of caregiving?* Paper presented at the annual meeting of the Gerontological Society, Chicago.

Manson, S. (1984). *Final report. Problematic life situations: Cross-cultural variation in support mobilization among the elderly.* Portland, OR: Institute on Aging, School of Urban and Public Affairs, Portland State University.

Matthews, S. (1995). Gender and the division of filial responsibility between lone sisters and their brothers. *Journal of Gerontology: Social Sciences, 50B,* S312–320.

McAdoo, H. (1998). African-American families. In C. Mindel, R. Habenstein, & R. Wright, Jr. (Eds.), *Ethnic families in America* (4th ed.) (pp. 361–381). Upper Saddle River, NJ: Prentice Hall.

McCallum, J., & Gelfand, D. (1990). *Ethnic women in the middle: A focus group study of daughters caring for older migrants in Australia.* Canberra, Australia: National Centre for Epidemiology and Population Health, Australian National University.

Merrill, D., & Dill, A. (1989, November). *Ethnic differences in family caregiving.* Paper presented at the annual meeting of the Gerontological Society of America, Minneapolis, MN.

Min, P. G. (1998). The Korean-American family. In C. Mindel, R. Habenstein, & R. Wright, Jr. (Eds.), *Ethnic families in America* (4th ed.) (pp. 223–253). Upper Saddle River, NJ: Prentice Hall.

Morioka-Douglas, N., & Yeo, G. (1990). *Aging and health: Asian-Pacific Island American elders.* Stanford, CA: Stanford Geriatric Education Center.

Ortega, W., Crutchfield, R., & Rushing, W. (1983). Race differences in elderly personal well-being. *Research on Aging, 5,* 101–118.

Polacca, M. (2001). American Indian and Alaska Native elderly. In L. Olson (Ed.), *Age through ethnic lenses: Caring for the elderly in a multicultural society* (pp. 113–122). Lanham, MD: Rowman and Littlefield.

Pruchno, R. (1999). Raising grandchildren: The experiences of Black and White grandmothers. *The Gerontologist, 39,* 209–221.

Red Horse, J., Lewis, R., Feit, M., & Decker, J. (1978). Family behavior of urban American Indians. *Social Casework, 59,* 67–72.

Rosenthal, C. (1986). Family supports in late life: Does ethnicity make a difference. *The Gerontologist, 26,* 19–24.

Sanchez-Ayendez, M. (1998). The Puerto Rican American family. In C. Mindel, R. Habenstein, & R. Wright, Jr. (Eds.), *Ethnic families in America: Patterns and variations* (4th ed.) (pp. 199–222). New York: Elsevier.

Smith, J. (1993). Function and supportive roles of church and religion. In J. Jackson, L. Chatters, & R. Taylor (Eds.), *Aging in Black America.* Newbury Park, CA: Sage.

Starrett, R., Sousa, D., Decker, J., Walter, G., & Keller, W. (n.d.). *The mental health behavior of the Hispanic elderly: A comparison of use of professional, physician and church.* Unpublished manuscript.

Stoller, E. (1987). Ethnicity in the informal networks of older sunbelt migrants: A case history of the Finns in Florida. In D. Gelfand & C. Barresi (Eds.), *Ethnic dimensions of aging* (pp. 118–129). New York: Springer Publishing.

Stoller, E. (1998). Informal exchanges with non-kin among retired sunbelt migrants: A case study of a Finnish American retirement community. *Journal of Gerontology: Social Sciences, 53B,* S287–S298.

Strawbridge, W., & Wallhagen, M. (1992). Is all in the family always best? *Journal of Aging Studies, 6,* 81–92.

Sue, G. (1989). Ethnic identity: The impact of two cultures on the psychological development of Asians in America. In D. Atkinson, G. Morten, & D. Wing (Eds.), *Counseling American minorities* (pp. 103–115). Dubuque, IA: William C. Brown.

Suarez, Z. (1998). Cuban-American families. In C. Mindel, R. Habenstein, & R. Wright, Jr. (Eds.), *Ethnic families in America: Patterns and variations* (4th ed.) (pp. 172–198). New York: Elsevier.

Talamantes, N., Cornell, J., Espino, D., Lichtenstein, H., & Hazuda, H. (1996). SES and ethnic differences in perceived caregiver availability among young-old Mexican Americans and non-Hispanic Whites. *The Gerontologist, 36,* 88–99.

Talamantes, M., Espino, D., Cornell, J., Lichtenstein, H., & Hazuda, H. (1992, November). *Caregiver availability and type among Mexican and non-Hispanic White young elderly.* Paper presented at the annual meeting of the Gerontological Society of America, Washington, DC.

Valle, R. (1983). The demography of Mexican American aging. In R. McNeely & J. Colen (Eds.), *Aging in minority groups.* Beverly Hills, CA: Sage.

Wallace, K., & Bergeman, C. (2001). *A cross-cultural examination of protective factors in minority elders.* Paper presented at the annual meeting of the Gerontological Society, Chicago, IL.

Weibel-Orlando, J., & Kramer, J. (1989). *Urban American Indian elders outreach project.* Los Angeles: County Area Agency on Aging, Department of Community and Senior Citizens Services.

White, T., Townsend, A., & Stephens, M. (2000). Comparisons of African American and White women in the parent care role. *The Gerontologist, 40,* 718–728.

Williams, G. (1980). Warriors no more: A study of the American Indian elderly. In C. L. Fry (Ed.), *Aging in culture and society* (pp. 101–111). New York: Praeger.

Wilmoth, J. (2001). Living arrangements among older immigrants in the United States. *The Gerontologist, 41,* 228–238.

Yeo, G. (1992, November). Paper presented at the symposium on *Elderly immigrants in the United States: A future perspective.* Washington, DC: Gerontological Society of America.

Yoo, S., & Sung, K. (1997). Elderly Koreans tendency to live independently from their adult children. *Journal of Cross Cultural Gerontology, 12,* 225–244.

Chapter Six

Reaching and Meeting Ethnic Aged Needs

Any effort to evaluate whether existing programs meet the needs of the ethnic aged requires an analytic framework, the concepts of which can then be applied as measurement standards. Primary among analytic concepts for programs and services is their *adequacy*, the ability of programs and services to meet the needs of the people for whom they are intended. *Equity* "is the principle that a policy should treat all people who are in the same circumstances in the same way. As such, it is the primary criterion of the fairness or justice of a policy" (Kutzik, n.d., p. 19). As Kutzik notes, what is being described in this definition is not equity for an individual, but "social equity," that is, equity for the group. Under social equity, there are variations in treatment for groups, depending on their circumstances.

Even if programs are adequate and equitable for all groups, they can work at cross-purposes with other efforts. The result is a lack of coherence, which can blunt the effectiveness of the program. *Coherence* refers to the extent to which one program effort meshes with other initiatives.

Programs also have less visible impacts, or *latent consequences*, not originally intended by their framers. The latent consequences of social welfare efforts are a consideration in program evaluation, but also require consideration during program planning stages.

STANDARDS AND PROGRAMS FOR THE AGED

Program Adequacy

Measurement of adequacy requires an agreed-upon standard for a target goal. Even with limited goals, existing programs and services for the

132

elderly fail to meet any test of adequacy. Measured against the federal poverty standard, Social Security provides some basic income for older retirees, but its average payments can only barely meet the goal of adequacy. Some older people with limited work records are eligible for the SSI program. Without state supplementation of the cash benefits and Food Stamps, the SSI payments are also an inadequate means of reaching the federal poverty standard.

Since its introduction in 1965, Medicare has guaranteed basic health care coverage for older persons, but there are still many gaps in Medicare coverage. Major health care expenditures, including medication, dental care, eyeglasses, and long-term care, receive only limited or no reimbursement through Medicare. Medicare has also failed to provide an adequate mechanism for controlling the inflationary costs of medical care for the older population and the country as a whole.

Program Equity

Determination of whether programs for older populations are equitable is more controversial. African American, Latino, Asian, Native American, and White elderly are all eligible for programs and services, as long as they meet the age criteria of specific programs (60 for OAA programs), have contributed the required amounts to the program (Social Security), or are below the income and/or asset limitations of the program (SSI or Medicaid).

Equitable distribution of program resources also requires consideration of the relative needs of each group. The economic and health needs of minority elderly in the United States are greater than the needs of their age peers from most European-based backgrounds. Social equity, therefore, dictates an unequal distribution of resources in order to assure equity. Advocacy groups for minority elderly have argued for many years that the shorter life expectancy of their populations should allow their older members to qualify for programs at an earlier age; for example, 55 rather than 60 for OAA programs. Because of the increased numbers of people who would be served, and the resultant costs, the federal government has resisted this change.

The issue of equity is also evident in the formulas that state governments use to distribute funds, which they receive from the Administration on Aging, to county and city government agencies that operate or coordinate programs for older persons. In 1987, a Florida court ruled that the intrastate funding formula was discriminatory, because it did not include any consideration of the number of minority elderly in the state. Many states have assumed that an intrastate funding formula that includes the percentage of elderly below the federal poverty level would guarantee an adequate representation of minority elderly. As a result of the Florida decision, new intrastate funding formulas are likely to contain both the percentage of older persons living below the poverty level and the percentage of minority elderly in the state's population.

Services are now often targeted to minority elderly, in order to ensure equitable representation in aging programs and services. As is true of the intrastate funding formula, targeting is an effort to ensure that resources are distributed equitably, based on considerations of need, particularly among minority elderly. Targeting requirements are now part of the OAA.

Program Coherence

Coherence among programs and services is sometimes difficult to obtain in the United States, because of the number of layers of government, involved in any effort. Even at one particular level of government coherence may be elusive. Efforts to cut taxes may be viewed as positive by older people. These tax reductions may not be coherent with cuts in Medicare to replace these lost revenues. The Medicare reductions may have more of an impact on less-affluent ethnic aged, who cannot compensate for the loss of Medicare coverage or reimbursement. In the same manner, mergers of organizations serving disparate geographic areas of a state, in order to save on administrative costs, is not necessarily coherent with a policy whose aim is to target programs for minority elderly living in a specific geographic area.

Latent Consequences of Programs

By definition, the latent consequences of a program are not readily apparent. A common assumption is that education about health problems will not only encourage individuals to seek better formal health care, but also to modify their health practices. Even the best-intentioned program, however, may have latent consequences that are negative in their outcome. Home-delivered meals are oriented to older people who cannot leave their homes. A possible latent consequence of these programs is their encouragement of older people to remain at home, rather than seek out environments that provide social interaction.

Major questions have also been raised about the extent to which the development of an extensive nursing home sector weakens family members' feelings of responsibility for community-based assistance for the aged. A good test of this possible latent consequence will be the development of nursing homes among Native American groups. Numbering less than 10 in 1990, nursing homes are a contrast to the clanbased system of care found among tribes such as the Navajo (Kunitz & Levy, 1991).

ISSUES IN SERVICE UTILIZATION

Adequacy, equity, coherence, and latent consequences are not the only issues to be considered in the evaluation of a program. Programs can be evaluated at many different levels, but much of this analysis concentrates on organizational issues. At the individual level, it is important to probe whether necessary programs and services exist and can be utilized by the ethnic aged person. One approach to this scrutiny of programs is the simple model of four A's: *availability, awareness, acceptability,* and *accessibility* of services (Fig. 6.1).

Service Availability

Availability refers to whether the basic programs and services needed by the ethnic elderly are being offered in the community. Availability

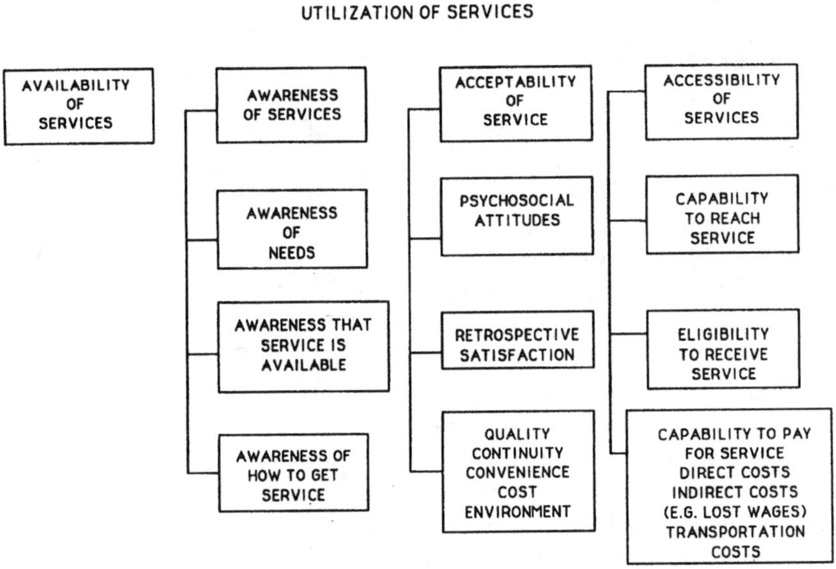

UTILIZATION OF SERVICES

FIGURE 6.1   Factors influencing service utilization by ethnic elderly.

cannot be measured simply by counting agency listings in the telephone book. A service that is open from 9 to 5 on weekdays may not really be available to many minority elderly who work during these hours. Insufficient funds make hiring sufficient staff difficult for many programs. Even though many others in the community need it, inadequate physical space may also limit the availability of the services to a small clientele. For the ethnic aged, there is the additional concern of locating staff who speak their language. Unavailability of bilingual staff may be a sufficient reason for Latino, Vietnamese, or Polish elderly to avoid participation in a senior center, or not to apply for entitlement programs that could improve their financial security.

Beyond lacking fluency in the languages of their clients, the agency staff may not have any understanding of ethnic cultures. Intentionally or unintentionally, they may violate important ethnic norms. Whatever the intentions of the staff, the older ethnic person may view staff behavior as symptomatic of a lack of respect.

Although a program or service may be available to older persons, it may not be available to all older persons. The programs and services authorized under the OAA are unique in this regard, since they are available to all persons over age 60. Other programs, such as Social Security, require a past contribution to the system. In the case of SSI, the older person must prove dire need. Poverty status is also required for eligibility for Medicaid.

Service Awareness

Awareness of services involves a number of levels on the part of the older consumer or potential consumer of services. These include an awareness of the need, an awareness that services are available to meet that need, and an awareness of how to obtain the appropriate service.

Many older individuals are potential consumers of a variety of programs and services. A number of important factors encourage them to become actual program and service users. One factor is their awareness of a need for programs and services. New health problems, a reduction in living conditions, or a loss of income may alert the older person to a need for some formal assistance.

In other cases, the older person who finds a means of coping with problems may deny the need for formal assistance. They may have problems preparing adequate meals, and so will alter their eating habits. Processed foods and foods that are simpler to prepare but are not as nutritious, may be substituted for more complex meals. Others may be able to utilize the help of relatives or friends in preparing meals or shopping and cleaning. As their needs increase, older individuals may turn to formal services, even if their preferences are for informal assistance from family members. The level of disability, rather than ethnicity, has been found to account for the use of formal services among African American, Puerto Rican, and White elderly (Tennstedt, Chang, & Delgado, 1998), and in overall comparisons of Latinos and Whites (Wallace, Levy-Storm, & Ferguson, 1995).

Attitudes about formal services are partly a reflection of resources available to the older person. In African American communities where older individuals are able to call upon friends and church members for assistance, the need for formal services may be less apparent. In Latino communities, the intertwined blood and nonblood-related individuals, who are often viewed as part of the family, may provide needed assistance. Older Koreans may live in a multigenerational household that substitutes for some of the efforts of formal providers. The demands of American society, however, may make these traditional patterns of care difficult to perform: "As Puerto Rican families continue to adapt to the changing socioeconomic context of life in the mainland U.S., we cannot assume that their familism will override social demands (challenges) from external sources" (Tennstedt et al., 1998, p. 194).

Corresponding to an awareness of need on the part of older individuals, there also must be an awareness of services. In Australia, Turkish women providing care for their parents did not know about a variety of home care and respite services that were available to them at no cost (McCallum & Gelfand, 1990). Ethnic elderly in the United States may know that services exist, but assume that these services are only for very limited populations. If involved with the ethnic culture, the older person may have some knowledge of ethnically based services, but little knowledge of public programs. This pattern was found among urban Native American elderly in Los Angeles (Weibel-Orlando & Kramer, 1989). Among Latino elderly, knowledge of services was the best predictor of use of social, health, and mental health services (Cox & Monk, 1990). The knowledge of formal services among Korean elderly in Los Angeles has been found to be minimal. Less than 1% of 223 Korean older respondents knew about long-term care management, in comparison to 30% of Whites. The program best known to Korean elderly was senior centers. Although 51% of these older persons had knowledge of these centers, this percentage was much lower than the 93% of the White respondents who knew about senior centers (Moon, Lubben, & Villa, 1998).

Although need has been found to be the primary determinant of health service usage, Irizarry (1988) found that need was not statistically related to the use of social services by Latino elderly in Cleveland. Social service users were more knowledgeable about services and greater users of services in general. Among a diverse Latino population, knowledge of services, as well as need, predicted use of services (Starrett, Wright, Mindel, & Tran, 1984). Examining African American, Latino, and White elderly in Michigan, Chapleski (1990) found knowledge of services to be the greatest predictor of usage. The differences between health and social service usage may relate to the discretionary nature of social services, as compared with nondiscretionary health service needs (Starrett, Decker, Araujo, & Walters, 1989).

Also, the older person may know about public services in general, but have no knowledge of specific services targeted for older persons. This latter situation was found in a study of older African American men in Baltimore (Chester, 1990). These men met regularly at local restaurants, shopping malls, and social clubs, but rarely, if ever, used formal services. Although they had knowledge of the general social and health services available, their knowledge of programs and services directed to older people was more limited. Even with the knowledge that services exist, the ethnic aged person may not know how to apply for these services, nor their eligibility requirements.

Acceptability of Services

Awareness of need and an understanding of how to apply for available services does not mean that the older person is going to use those services. Traditions and psychosocial attitudes about the meaning of service utilization may discourage older people from obtaining the help they need. For many, these psychosocial attitudes hark back to negative feelings about accepting charity. The antipathy toward charity is likely to have great strength among ethnic elderly from a first-generation immigrant cohort. Proud of their survival and success in their new country, these older persons from Latino, European, or Asian backgrounds may view services as a reflection of inadequacy on their part. Antipathy toward services is also evident among older Black men and women who take pride in their ability to overcome discrimination and poor living conditions through their own resources.

Except for Social Security and OAA programs, most American programs are means tested. Eligibility for these programs requires individuals to prove their income is below a specific eligibility level. For foreign-born and American-born ethnic elderly, means testing may promote the view that programs and services are charity, and an indication that these individuals are no longer able to provide for themselves.

Cost sharing is now permitted with OAA programs. Under cost sharing, older persons can be asked to pay a portion of the costs of the program. At this time, the amount the older person contributes will be based solely on their declaration of their current income. Critics have argued that cost sharing will eventually include not only a declaration of income by the older person, but a full assessment of income and assets, including property, stocks, bonds, and other sources of income. It is unclear whether cost sharing will avoid the stigma of charity associated with means testing.

Ethnic aged who grew up in other countries have a variety of experiences with formal programs and services. In most Western European countries, formal services are extensive and accepted as part of everyday life. In Eastern European countries, the government has controlled formal services. The American model of voluntary agencies has not existed in Eastern Europe. In African and Latin American countries, formal services vary in their extensiveness and requirements. Many of the current cohort of American-born ethnic aged had their first encounter with programs and services run by the federal government during the Great Depression of the 1930s.

The depression reinforced the belief that the family and ethnic group always needed to be prepared to take care of their own. Italians and other European groups brought these attitudes with them from the old country. Cohler (1984) traces the high expectations of assistance from family and friends among Italians to traditional suspicions of formal organizations.

Among minority elderly, negative attitudes about government programs may be based on past discriminatory experiences. Although the federal government's intervention was important for many groups during the depression, discrimination occurred at both local and national levels. The Civilian Conservation Corps, for example, restricted enrollment of young African Americans to a maximum of 10% of the enrollees. Until 1947, the Federal Housing Administration also restricted home loans to minorities. Experiences such as these have naturally led to skepticism on the part of older African Americans about the commitment of government programs to meeting their needs.

One of the most widely discussed factors in mistrust of health and social services among African Americans is the infamous Tuskegee experiment, which studied the course of syphilis among Black men, by not informing or treating them for the disease. The Tuskegee experiment is perhaps the most widely cited case of exploitation of African Americans for health research, but it is not the only one: "Given a history that runs from experimentation on slaves to public health efforts gone awry in sickle cell screening and involuntary sterilization, conspiracy theories cannot be simply written off as paranoia or hypersensitivity" (Corbie-Smith & Arriola, 2001, p. 492).

Access to Services

For many people, *access* brings to mind the ability to reach a senior center or adult day care center with an automobile or by public transit. This view of access is too limited: It also means being able to climb the stairs at a school where a program is located, or being able to climb the steps of a bus to go to the program. Even if the older person is able to climb the bus steps, they may have difficulty affording the fare. The cost of reaching or using programs is also an important part of access.

Access to services can be made more or less difficult for individuals by the application or intake process. A complex set of application forms and interviews may restrict access to programs among fearful or less-educated ethnic elderly. Multiple-page application forms are part of such programs as SSI because of the complex eligibility requirements imposed on applicants. Even if they meet the income and asset standards of a program, the required tests and documentation frightens some older people away from services they desperately need. Fear of application forms may be intense among older people who do not have legal immigration status and who are worried about being identified and deported.

In some cases, eligibility to receive services may mean that the individual does not have to pay any fee. In other cases, however, the client may have to contribute a share of the costs. A 20% share of the costs, as in Medicare Part B, may be too onerous for the potential client to bear. Besides these direct costs, there are often indirect costs associated with programs. One possible cost is the loss of pay that may result if time off from work is used for a doctor's visit, or if someone has to be paid to provide child care for children or grandchildren.

Transportation is a major cost factor in service delivery. If, for example, the older person cannot afford the cost of regular taxicab rides, a reluctant decision may be made to use any mass transit that is available. In many cases, the existing services may be public buses. The financial costs of using a bus may be less than a taxicab, but a 30-minute trip by car may turn out to be a 90-minute bus ride, because of required transfers and waiting times between buses. Experiences of this kind are bound to discourage the use of programs and services, except in cases of stringent need.

Through Medicaid, very poor elderly may utilize services they cannot afford, even with Medicare coverage. Strict income limits, however, restrict the number of older people receiving Medicaid (although any older person receiving SSI qualifies for Medicaid). States administer and contribute extensively to Medicaid. Coverage beyond the basic services required by the federal government thus varies according to the relative financial prosperity or political climate of a particular state.

The net result of these factors, both singularly and in combination, is the underrepresentation of the ethnic aged in service usage, which occurs both in health care and in community-based services. In 1997, 10.7% of older persons using the community-based programs and services offered through the OAA were African American, 7.6% were Latino, 1.3% were American Indian/Native Alaskan, and 2.2% were Asian American/Pacific Islander (Administration on Aging, n.d.). These figures do not adequately represent the relative needs of older person in each of these four groups.

ETHNIC FACTORS IN SERVICE DELIVERY

At the individual and community level, there are many issues that hamper the utilization of programs and services by older people. Beyond the general issues already described, however, there are factors specific to ethnic populations, which play a role in determining service usage. These factors include:

1. lack of knowledge on the part of the ethnic aged about cultures other than their own
2. stereotypes among the ethnic aged about other ethnic groups
3. lack of knowledge among the ethnic aged of available services
4. unwillingness of the ethnic aged to travel beyond certain defined neighborhood boundaries
5. low expectation of services on the part of the ethnic aged
6. strong preferences among the ethnic aged for the maintenance of ethnic culture

Lack of Knowledge of Other Cultures

The growth in diversity among the ethnic population has also been accompanied by diversity in housing situations. As the history of migration indicates, ethnic groups usually settle in a particular neighborhood where other individuals of the same ethnic background reside. A common residential area helps families cope with a new environment, without immediately having to learn a new language or new customs. Stores catering to the food and clothing preferences of the residents are important anchors in these neighborhoods. As members of this ethnic community become acculturated and accumulate more resources, they move to an area of second settlement, where better housing and amenities exist.

By the time a second, third, and even fourth generation of this ethnic group exists, there may be both homogeneous ethnic communities and communities that are heterogeneous in their ethnic makeup. In the past, heterogeneous communities have represented more-affluent areas and the homogeneous communities poorer, inner-city areas. More recently, the migration of Whites from neighborhoods, as minority families have moved in, has resulted in the growth of middle-class ethnic communities in suburbia. Monterey Park, California, has the distinction of being the first Asian suburb in the United States. Prince Georges County, Maryland, has many communities comprised of middle-class African American families. Increased segregation of ethnic neighborhoods in inner-city and suburban areas is a trend that reduces the possibility of interethnic contacts.

The ethnic neighborhood has important advantages for many individuals, such as solidarity and a sense of belonging to a vital culture, but the disadvantages should also be noted. Living in an ethnic neighborhood may, unfortunately, promote a "we–they" feeling. Individuals who do not belong to the same ethnic group are seen, at best, as outsiders. At its worst, this ethnocentric attitude promotes a feeling that people from other ethnic backgrounds are threats, and that contact with "them" should be avoided to the greatest extent possible. In periods of poor economic growth, the we–they feeling may increase. During these times, other ethnic groups may become the scapegoat for problems facing the ethnic group. High-density homogeneous ethnic neighborhoods may restrict the contact an individual has with other ethnic cultures. Institutional completeness may reinforce that isolation, since the ethnic group does not have to rely on outside resources to provide education or health services.

If positive attitudes about other cultures exist, and there is an absence of entrenched stereotypes, contact among ethnic groups can be an important step toward improving intercultural relations. This contact, however, must be on the basis of equality between the groups, rather than one group's superiority to the other. For example, the only contact that many African American aged have with Jews has been with Jewish storeowners in the African American community. These Jewish merchants were seen as exploitative and usurious. As Jews have moved into the professions, Asians have become owners of many of the small stores in African American communities. African Americans in New York and Washington, DC, have reacted passionately to reported maltreatment of African American customers by Korean storeowners and their supposed unwillingness to hire African Americans as employees. In Detroit, tensions between Arab storeowners and African Americans have at times erupted into violence.

The contact of many Whites with Latinos has been limited to Latinos who work as domestics in private homes or hotels, or perhaps as agricultural workers. Even more limited is the contact of Whites with Native Americans. These contacts are confined to some major cities with non-reservation Indian workers or to areas where there are substantial Native American populations.

Interethnic contact based on unequal status does not guarantee a greater understanding or more positive attitude toward other cultures. A lack of interethnic contact, however, can be equally important in creating barriers that prevent the development of important programmatic changes. Lukas (1985) demonstrates how a lack of interethnic contact and understanding amplified the hostilities between African Americans and Irish in Boston, as school busing began in the 1970s.

Stereotypes of Ethnic Groups

The attitudes ethnic aged bring into their later years have developed during earlier periods of their residence in the United States or other countries. These attitudes may have hardened into stereotypes. Stereotypes are prevalent about many ethnic groups, and it is illuminating to observe how stereotypes change or remain stable over time. Radio, television, and film have only recently begun to scrutinize the images of the Native Americans, African Americans, Asians, and Latinos that they present.

Stereotypes of African Americans have changed dramatically during the twentieth century. African Americans, particularly men, are no longer portrayed as lovable, but uneducated. Instead, they may be viewed as threatening and violent. Latino stereotypes still emphasize the lazy Mexican. Stereotypes of White ethnic groups have become less clear over time, as these groups have become more integrated into American society and less distinct in their lifestyles. However, the Irish drunk, the Jewish banker, and the Italian gangster remain prevalent in the American consciousness. One of the newest and most negative stereotypes is that of dirty, "shifty," and dangerous Arabs. This stereotype was reinforced in 2001 by the destruction of the World Trade Center in New York.

Ethnic groups may also be portrayed in positive stereotypes, such as the recent stereotype of Asians. But these may also be damaging to the group. Stereotypes of Asians have changed from those warning of the "yellow peril" to those portraying Asians as respectful, studious, and without any problems. Spokespeople for Asian groups now have to battle against the "model minority" stereotype, which often mitigates against Asians receiving the programs and services they need.

The ethnic aged are affected by two stereotypes: the stereotype of their specific ethnic group and the stereotype of the elderly, which is prevalent in American society. Ironically, there seem to be two dichotomous stereotypes about older people current in American society. The first stereotype has been prevalent for many years and portrays older individuals as feeble, doting, and cognitively impaired. The second, more recent stereotype portrays older people as high-income individuals who spend their time traveling and catering to their desires, without any concern for the needs of younger individuals. This latter stereotype has often been labeled the "greedy geezer" stereotype. Acceptance of the first stereotype makes it difficult for older people to maintain important roles in society, since they are viewed as impaired. Acceptance of the second stereotype ignores the problems of lower income and frailer older individuals. The stereotype contributes to the difficulty of obtaining programs and services for these needy individuals.

Applied on a societal level, stereotypes are important in determining an individual's opportunities for advancement. Accepted stereotypes play a role in determining how a person feels about associating with other ethnic groups. Societal stereotypes of the aged, as either feeble or wealthy and selfish, feed back into relative levels of support for public funding of programs and services. Individual acceptance of ethnic stereotypes may influence an older person's willingness to participate in organizations with other ethnic aged.

More educated, better trained, second- and third-generation ethnic individuals have had increased opportunity to interact with other ethnic groups on an equal basis. This has been especially true in the last 30 years. As the baby boom generation ages, there will be increased numbers of ethnic aged people who have had varied interethnic experiences in their general interactions and in their work relationships. High rates of intermarriage, by groups such as Japanese Americans (Kitano &

Kitano, 1998), will also alter attitudes about ethnic groups. The continuation of residential segregation by ethnicity and class will have the opposite effect. Residential segregation will limit the possibility of interethnic contacts among school-age children and reinforce negative ethnic stereotypes (Marano & Bravo, 2002).

Fear, mistrust, hostility, or stereotypic images of other ethnic groups are factors that often need to be overcome to obtain the participation of the ethnic aged with other ethnic groups. The same feelings may also extend to the older person's dealings with professionals. The older person may mistrust professionals from other ethnic backgrounds. Language barriers, including limited English on the part of the older client or the provider, add to the potential for misunderstandings. Ethnic aged who do not welcome, or who feel unwelcomed, by other ethnic groups may request separate services. Few organizations have the facilities to provide separate physical space for each ethnic group in their service-delivery area, or the funds to hire staff to match the ethnic background of the aged. Among recent immigrant groups, there are often only a few individuals with professional service-delivery backgrounds. Even in an area with a large Cuban population, such as South Florida, finding qualified bilingual individuals, who can communicate effectively with older individuals, is not always easy (Marano & Bravo, 2002).

There is no simple solution to this dilemma. Changing people's attitudes about race and ethnicity has been found to be more difficult than changing behaviors. Placed in contact with persons from other ethnic groups, older individuals may accommodate these other groups, even if their attitudes and stereotypes remain intact. Over time, these attitudes and stereotypes may change.

Lack of Knowledge of Available Services

Guttmann (1979) attributes the low service-utilization rate of ethnic aged Whites to lack of knowledge of what services are available. Ignorance of services is also a problem among other groups. Limited fluency in English may account for some of the lack of knowledge of programs and services among Latino and Asian populations. Some populations may not even be literate in their mother tongue. Inability to read or write Spanish means that flyers and brochures cannot be used to communicate information about services to some older Latinos.

It is easy, but incorrect, to totally blame a lack of knowledge about programs and services on the older individual. In some communities, an ignorance of services may reflect disinterest on the part of service providers. Providers may be prejudiced against a particular group, or accept stereotypes that a specific group has problems beyond the capacity of any organization. Because of choice and discrimination, African Americans and Native Americans have established a tradition of "taking care of their own" through informal care arrangements. This history may lead to a perception among providers that these groups are not interested in any formal programs or services.

Because of the problems in obtaining funding for programs and services, providers may also be less attentive to lower-income communities, where the ability to pay for services is limited. Some providers deliberately avoid publicity about their programs, because they fear creating a demand for services that they cannot meet because of limited funds or staff.

Unwillingness to Travel to Services

For the individual entrenched in the local ethnic community, the outside world may be any location not in the immediate neighborhood. "Outside" may be threatening merely because it is unfamiliar. This outside world may also be threatening because it contains individuals who are "different." Fear of the larger environment may be heightened among individuals whose knowledge of English is limited, who have difficulty reading signs, or whose physical strength and ambulatory ability are limited. Therefore, it should not be surprising that an Italian woman in her eighties expresses concerns about attending a program or going to a medical clinic in another community, particularly if she has no familiarity with the subway or bus system or finds the high steps of the bus difficult to climb. Language problems among Latino and Asian elderly may make the outside community even more frightening and inaccessible.

Problems in walking or using public transportation often result in older people defining their neighborhood as a smaller physical unit than do younger individuals. Venturing outside this limited neighborhood, into areas populated by other ethnic groups, may be more threatening to the older ethnic person than to their younger counterparts.

Low Expectation of Services

For many ethnic older persons, past experiences with services have been unsatisfactory. The seemingly endless bureaucratic maze that often seems to be intrinsic to human services can be confusing to anyone, but the forms and rules are even more confusing for older individuals with limited education or fluency in English. Hearing and vision problems, as well as minimal access to transportation, reinforce decisions not to utilize services. The eligibility forms used by many programs and services may be necessary, but they are often combined with an impersonal approach that is anathema to many older people. Being called by a number and treated as a "case" does not help to reinforce older people's feelings that their needs are really the concern of the service provider.

Health and human service providers are often overburdened by large caseloads and limited resources. Providers may therefore adopt a view that the recipients of services should be deserving and grateful. Workers often find the special attention required by limited English-speaking ethnic aged to be frustrating and time-consuming. Faced with bureaucratic regulations and disconcerted by the impatience or indifference of service providers, older adults may conclude that they cannot expect to obtain any quality services. In turn, service providers who are genuinely concerned about senior citizens find the low service expectations of many ethnic aged an obstacle to obtaining high levels of program participation.

Effective Outreach

Maximizing appropriate service usage requires effective outreach. Although its importance has been recognized, effective outreach to the ethnic aged has been limited. For example, health-promotion literature recognizes the importance of differences among the ethnic aged (Fallcreek & Franks, 1984), but fails to provide substantial advice about techniques that are needed for effective health promotion with different ethnic groups. It is thus difficult to determine whether a therapeutic health program (Husaini et al., 1990), which proves to be effective with African American elderly, would be equally effective, without revision, for elderly from other ethnic backgrounds.

Yeatts and Crow (1990) have summarized outreach techniques for minority elderly stressed in the literature. Their review can be divided into "information techniques" and the "creation of positive attitudes." Yeatts and Crow demonstrate that there are many forms of media communication available for reaching the minority elderly. These include flyers and brochures, advertisements in the Yellow Pages, and television and radio. In many cases, radio and television may be more appropriate mechanisms for reaching older Latinos. Ramirez et al. (1983) report positive effects from using short radio novellas to communicate important information about heart disease to older Latinos. The novellas are five minutes long and have five episodes. Each episode discusses a risk factor in cardiovascular disease and how it could be prevented. Posttests indicated that the novella effectively communicated the desired information and that 39% of the 75 respondents took some action based on the information they obtained from the novellas. In their use of the novellas, the program developers built upon the strong interest of many Latinos in soap operas and radio dramas.

Even more effective than radio communication can be the use of significant individuals (Yeatts & Crow, 1990). Besides the relatives and friends of the older person, community organization leaders, site managers in elderly housing complexes, and school children are potential transmitters of important communications. The notes that children bring home from school can be an effective means of informing grandparents about programs that are available. Flyers at supermarkets and other stores are also possible sites for communicating information.

More importantly, there may be gathering places for older people in many communities. These gathering places are not necessarily senior centers. In a small study in Maryland, older African American men were found to congregate in restaurants and social clubs in their neighborhood, while ignoring the availability of senior centers (Chester, 1990). Proprietors and managers of these clubs can be purveyors of information.

One overall approach to outreach to minority populations in general has been termed the *community-based diffusion model* (National Heart, Lung, and Blood Institute [NHLBI], 1987). As shown in Figure 6.2, a number of different communication channels are viewed as appropriate for different minority populations. These variations relate to the socioeconomic, residential, and organizational patterns of the respective groups. Church leaders are important channels of communication for all the groups, hairdressers are valued for African Americans, and senior centers for all groups except Latinos. As more Latinos join senior centers, the importance of these organizations as communication channels may increase. Store proprietors are not vital in the communication chain for African Americans or Native Americans, because of the limited number of proprietors from these ethnic groups.

Religious leaders may also be important individuals in the outreach efforts. Among African Americans, the enlistment of ministers was found to be important in convincing African American men of the importance of prostate cancer screening (Powell, Gelfand, Parzuchowski, Heil-

COMMUNITY COMMUNICATION CHANNELS	AMERICAN INDIAN	ASIAN PACIFIC	BLACK	HISPANIC
Family, general	X	X	X	X
Children	X	X	X	X
Hairdressers/barbers			X	·
Sheriff/police dept.			X	
Church leaders	X	X	X	X
"Public" nurses	X	X	X	X
Social workers	X	X	X	X
Cinema owners/operators				X
Store proprietors		X		X
Professional organizations	X	X	X	X
Senior centers	X	X	X	
Work crew leaders			X	X
"Ethnic" newspapers	X	X		X
Political leaders	X	X	X	
Women's church groups	X	X	X	X
Television/radio	X	X	X	X
Mainstream health workers	X	X	X	X
Friends/peers	X	X	X	
Social/cultural clubs	X	X	X	X

FIGURE 6.2 Examples of communication channels utilized by the elderly.

Source: National Heart, Lung, and Blood Institute, 1987.

bron, & Franklin, 1995). Asked about their willingness to utilize palliative care programs such as hospice, Mexicans in Michigan and Arizona felt that endorsement of these services by a Catholic priest would be important to the community (Gelfand, Balcazar, Parzuchowski, & Lenox, 2001).

Obstacles to Effective Outreach

The most well-designed health promotion project may not be effective if older people reject the idea of changes in their health habits. Older persons may reject health advice because it conflicts with their own health norms or because they believe it is wrong to try to prolong life past a certain age. As an older Korean woman commented about medicines: "Why should old people take those to live longer? I prefer to live just the life span which was given to me. It is shameful, greedy, and ugly to live a long time. When the time comes, we have to die naturally" (Pang, 1991, p. 15).

Outreach Themes

The ethnic aged person may also reject changes because the "message" was not correctly oriented to cultural values. The community-based diffusion model suggests that certain themes are more readily accepted by some minority populations than others. Native Americans are viewed as less likely to respond to health messages based on fear, since this group is accustomed to "living with fear" (NHLBI, 1987). Instead, "love of family," "maintaining independence," or "remaining strong" are the most persuasive themes for Native Americans (p. 14). In contrast, Latinos will be more responsive to fear messages, particularly if they emphasize possible death or disability and include concerns about surviving children.

Love of family is presented as a theme valuable for both Latinos and Asian/Pacific Islanders. Among Asians, a theme stressing fear of dependency (NHLBI, p. 14) can also be utilized, if not overdone. Whatever the themes utilized for Asians/Pacific Islanders, they must take into account attitudes that stress the importance of self-sufficiency, self-control as a remedy, and fatalism. These values are positive factors in the ability of Asians/Pacific Islanders to achieve socioeconomic success and social mobility, but they often restrict the willingness of these groups to utilize formal services.

Effective outreach in African American communities has utilized a message that stresses the theme "Do it for your loved ones." Although this theme can be accompanied by fear messages, the fears must not be overstated and remedies to the fears raised in the messages must be suggested. The NHLBI also notes that, "Logical approaches, such as 'You take care of your shoes, you take care of your car, so take care of yourself,' may work as well" (p. 14).

These suggestions are enticing, because they appear to be specific to various ethnic groups, but they cannot be regarded as more than clues to the type of outreach approach that could prove effective with a particular racial/ethnic population. Whether the approach suggested for each group will be equally effective with older persons within these groups is not yet clear.

Personal communication may be very effective with minority and ethnic elderly who are skeptical about the value of specific programs and services. When asked why they came, senior center participants in

Maryland (Gelfand, Bechill, & Chester, 1990) stressed the personal communication they had from current participants. Using current program participants in a door-to-door canvassing effort, particularly in the participants' own neighborhoods, has some of the effects of a personal endorsement. All of these techniques assume the availability of services that are accessible to the older person and meet the needs of the older person, in a culturally acceptable manner.

The effectiveness of personal communication reinforces the view that the credentials of the person delivering an outreach message are often as important as the message itself. This has recently been confirmed in a prostate cancer outreach program targeted at older African American men in Detroit. African American men have the highest incidence of prostate cancer of any population in the world and have three times the mortality rate of American Whites. Unfortunately, national public screenings for prostate cancer have failed to secure high rates of participation by African American men. The Detroit outreach effort utilized a pool of African American men who had been treated successfully for prostate cancer. These prostate cancer survivors collaborated with a health professional to deliver educational programs about prostate cancer to African American men in churches throughout the community. Physicians and nurses have superior technical knowledge of prostate cancer, but the cancer survivors' appearances before other men indicated that prostate cancer can be detected and treated successfully. The fear that any form of cancer is an automatic death sentence was thus laid to rest (Powell et al., 1995).

The diversity of the ethnic population, including the presence of second-, third-, and even fourth-generation individuals among many groups, means that outreach approaches must be diverse. Undertaking outreach targeted for all the ethnic elderly, not only to the older individuals within the particular group, may also be most effective. For groups that are unfamiliar with the American system of voluntary agencies and health care, outreach for the older person may be more effectively targeted at their older individual's children or other more acculturated individuals. For these efforts, English language newspapers and media may be effective.

The appropriateness of different outreach approaches may also depend on the attitudes of ethnic populations. Rodriguez (2001) has argued that Latinos are developing a different pattern of acculturation in the United States than other minorities. There are no Latino-oriented universities and the Spanish language television stations are mainly utilized by first-generation immigrants. Intermarriage rates among Latinos and non-Latinos are high and expected to increase. Based on this analysis, outreach in Latino communities needs to be broad-based and include a variety of approaches, media, and social institutions.

In some cultures, outreach can also utilize what could be termed *culture carriers* (Michigan Partnership for the Advancement of End-of-Life Care, n.d.). This term was used by Native Americans in a recent research project focused on diffusion of end-of-life information. In the Native American community, culture carriers may be elders or individuals with a strong involvement in the traditional culture. Other cultures may have culture carriers who are community leaders. Although many of these cultural carriers may have formal positions in the group as ministers, tribal leaders and other culture carriers may not have any formally recognized role. They may, however, be well known in the community. Discovering who these community leaders are and their role in the community can be a first step in successful diffusion of information to ethnic elderly. Support of these culture carriers and community leaders can also be a major boost in gaining legitimacy for the outreach efforts. Legitimacy is particularly important if the outreach effort is being mounted by an organization that is not ethnically based, such as a health care program or even an aging organization.

Overcoming all of the hurdles to an adequate, equitable, and accessible system of programs and services that ethnic aged will want to use, and will be able to utilize, is the first part of a difficult task. The second part is the design of specific programs and services that address the needs of older people in general, and the ethnic aged in particular. The programs and services that now exist, and their relevance to the ethnic aged, are examined in Chapter 7.

References

Administration on Aging. (n.d.). 1997 state performance reports: *Table 3. Minority persons served under Title III of OAA: FY 1997.* Retrieved May 27, 2002, from *http://www.aoa.dhhs.gov/napis/97spr/tables/table2.html*

Chapleski, E. (1990, November). *Determinants of utilization of services to the elderly: A political economy perspective.* Paper presented at the Gerontological Society of America, Boston.

Chester, R. (1990). *Health and social services utilization among older Black males: A pilot study.* Baltimore: School of Social Work, University of Maryland at Baltimore.

Cohler, B. (1984). Europeans. In E. Palmore (Ed.), *Handbook of the aged in the United States* (pp. 235–252). Westport, CT: Greenwood Press.

Corbie-Smith, G., & Arriola, K. (2001). Research and ethics. In R. Braithwaite & S. Taylor (Eds.), *Health issues in the Black community* (2nd ed., pp. 489–502). San Francisco: Jossey-Bass.

Cox, C., & Monk, A. (1990). Minority caregivers of dementia victims: A comparison of Black 'and Hispanic families. *Journal of Applied Gerontology, 9,* 340–354.

Fallcreek, S., & Franks, J. (1984). *Health promotion and aging.* Washington, DC: Department of Health and Human Services.

Gelfand, D., Balcazar, H., Parzuchowski, J., & Lenox, S. (2001). Information and services in end-of-life care for Latinos: The role of media, family, church and hospice. *American Journal of Hospice and Palliative Care, 18,* 391–396.

Gelfand, D., Bechill, W., & Chester, R. (1990). *Maryland senior centers: Programs, services and linkages.* Baltimore: School of Social Work, University of Maryland at Baltimore.

Guttmann, D. (1979). Use of informal and formal support by White ethnic aged. In D. Gelfand & A. Kutzik (Eds.), *Ethnicity and aging: Theory, research, and policy* (pp. 246–262). New York: Springer Publishing.

Husaini, B., Castor, R., Whitten-Stovall, R., Moore, S., Neser, W., Linn, J. G., et al. (1990). An evaluation of the therapeutic health program for the black elderly. *Journal of Health and Social Policy, 2,* 67–85.

Irizarry, A, (1988). *Knowledge and utilization of social services among the Hispanic elderly.* Final Report, Applied Gerontological Fellowship. Washington, DC: Gerontological Society of America.

Kitano, K., & Kitano, H. (1998). The Japanese-American family. In C. Mindel, R. Habenstein, & R. Wright, Jr. (Eds.), *Ethnic families in America: Patterns and variations* (4th ed.) (pp. 311–330). New York: Elsevier.

Kunitz, S., & Levy, J. (1991). *Navajo aging.* Tucson, AZ: University of Arizona Press.

Kutzik, A. (n.d.). Equity. In *Conceptual tools.* Baltimore: School of Social Work, University of Maryland at Baltimore.

Lukas, J. (1985). *Common ground.* New York: Alfred A. Knopf.

Marano, C., & Bravo, M. (2002). A psychoeducational model for Hispanic Alzheimer's disease caregivers. *The Gerontologist, 42,* 122–126.

McCallum, J., & Gelfand, D. (1990). *Ethnic women in the middle: A focus group study of daughters caring for older migrants in Australia.* Canberra, Australia: National Centre for Epidemiology and Population Health, Australian National University

Michigan Partnership for the Advancement of End-of-Life Care (n.d.). *How do community members seek information about end-of-life care?* Report from the Community Resources Project Team. Lansing, MI: Author.

Moon, A., Lubben, J., & Villa, V. (1998). Awareness and utilization of community long-term care services by elderly Korean and non-Hispanic White Americans. *The Gerontologist, 38,* 309–316.

National Heart, Lung, and Blood Institute. (1987). *Executive Summary: Strategies for diffusing health information to minority populations.* Washington, DC: Author.

Pang, K. (1991). *Korean elderly women in America: Everyday life, health and illness.* New York: AMS Press.

Powell, S., Gelfand, D., Parzuchowski, J., Heilbron, L., & Franklin, A. (1995). A successful recruitment process of African American men for early detection of prostate cancer. *Cancer, 75*(7) (Suppl.), 1880–1884.

Ramirez, A., Santos, Y., Slayton, P., Gill, S., Britt, R., & Cousins, J. (1983). *VIVIR O MORIR: The effects of radio on health education for Hispanics.* Paper presented at the American Public Health Association, Dallas, TX.

Rodriguez, G. (2001, February 11). Mexican-Americans: Forging a new vision of America's melting pot. *New York Times,* 4:1, 4.

Starrett, R., Decker, J., Araujo, A., & Walters, G. (1989). The Cuban elderly and their service use. *Journal of Applied Gerontology, 8,* 69–85.

Starrett, R., Wright, R., Mindel, C., & Tran, T. (1984). The use of social services by Hispanic elderly: A comparison of Mexican-Americans, Puerto Rican and Cuban elderly. *Journal of Social Services Research, 13,* 1–26.

Tennstedt, S., Chang, B.-H., & Delgado, M. (1998). Patterns of long-term care: A comparison of Puerto Rican, African American and non-Latino White elderly. *Journal of Gerontological Social Work, 30*(1/2), 179–199.

Wallace, S., Levy-Storm, L., & Ferguson, L. (1995). Access to paid in-home assistance among disabled elderly people: Do Latinos differ from non-Latino Whites. *American Journal of Public Health, 85,* 970–975.

Weibel-Orlando, J., & Kramer, J. (1989). *Urban American Indian elders outreach project.* Los Angeles: Los Angeles County Area Agency on Aging, Department of Community and Senior Citizens Services.

Yeatts, D., & Crow, T. (1990). *Practical techniques for attracting the low-income minority elderly to area agency services.* Washington, DC: Fellowship Program in Applied Gerontology, Gerontological Society of America.

Chapter Seven

Programs, Services, and the Ethnic Aged

As Markides, Liang, and Jackson (1990) point out, many minority elderly enter old age with inadequate resources. Discrimination in education, jobs, and housing, and the limited availability of health and social services, presage a difficult time for the older African American, Latino, Asian, or Native American. Immigrant status creates additional problems. Cultural differences, language barriers, and, if the individual is an illegal immigrant, ineligibility for important public services, impede successful aging. A group can also be denied services if they do not clearly fall into one specific ethnic category. For example, the Yaqui Indians, who are indigenous to Mexico, have often been denied services in the United States, because the Bureau of Indian Affairs considered them to be Mexicans (Aleman & Paz, 1998).

Elimination of problems that face the ethnic and minority aged requires not only adequate income maintenance programs and health care services, but also a complex of social and housing programs and services. Since the mid-1970s, the complex of services available for older persons has increased dramatically across the United States. Until recently, little, if any, consideration has been given to the approaches that would be most effective among the ethnic elderly.

ETHNOSPECIFIC PROGRAMS AND SERVICES

The existence of ethnic groups within a society does not automatically imply an acceptance of the need for separate services for all ethnic elderly. The limitations on ethnospecific services derive from both ideology and logistics. An effort to develop separate services for each group of minority elderly and ethnic aged in the United States is a daunting task. In midwestern and eastern metropolitan areas, this would mean separate services for groups that range from Albanians to Serbs, each with a valid claim to a distinct cultural identity and past.

Ideologically, ethnospecific services revive the controversy over the pluralistic versus assimilative nature of American society. A pluralistic, or multicultural, model of society allows for diversity. Separate facilities can be seen as one extreme of diversity. One objection to this separation is that, if all ethnic groups subscribe to a common core of American values, it should be possible for ethnic groups to share common facilities. This positive attitude often simplifies the long-standing hostilities that have existed among ethnic groups. If these histories are overlooked, ethnic hostilities may impede programming. The desire for specific ethnic foods, as well as programming oriented toward specific ethnic cultures, also fosters a desire among ethnic groups for separate programs and facilities.

The net result of current thinking is a paucity of programs and services targeted toward the ethnic elderly, except for limited efforts directed at minority elderly. Programs offered in neighborhoods where one ethnic group predominates are de facto oriented to the needs of this specific population. In most cases, ethnic elderly utilize the services offered under a variety of legislative auspices, as well as those programs and services offered through the so-called "aging network." This complex network of services is difficult to describe simply, and it may be confusing to the older person and their family. To clarify some of this confusion, it is necessary to examine the general services that are available to older people, as well as services specifically oriented to an older population.

The examination focuses on services as they now exist in the United States and on the possible revisions that would enable them to more effectively meet the needs of ethnic elderly. Specific programs and services for the older person include opportunities for socializing and special efforts devoted to the functional needs of older people. It is important, however, not to neglect the less obvious opportunities for ethnicity to play a role in general health and mental health programs and services. These programs are examined separately.

CONTINUUM OF CARE

The continuum of care is often utilized to classify services for the aged in the United States. Figure 7.1 is one graphic illustration of this

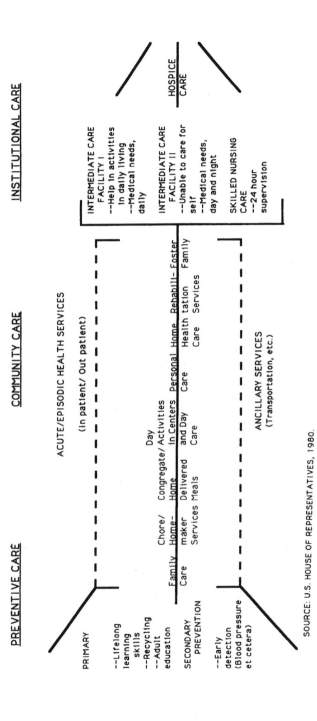

FIGURE 7.1 The continuum of care and its services for the aged.

PREVENTIVE CARE   COMMUNITY CARE   INSTITUTIONAL CARE

PRIMARY
--Lifelong learning skills
--Recycling
--Adult education

SECONDARY PREVENTION
--Early detection (Blood pressure et cetera)

ACUTE/EPISODIC HEALTH SERVICES
(In patient/ Out patient)

Family Home — Chore/ maker Services | Home Delivered Meals | Congregate/ Day Care | Activities In Centers and Day Care | Personal Care | Home Health Care | Rehabili- tation | Foster Family Services

ANCILLARY SERVICES
(Transportation, etc.)

INTERMEDIATE CARE FACILITY I
--Help in activities in daily living
--Medical needs, daily

INTERMEDIATE CARE FACILITY II
--Unable to care for self
--Medical needs, day and night

SKILLED NURSING CARE
--24 hour supervision

HOSPICE CARE

SOURCE: U.S. HOUSE OF REPRESENTATIVES, 1980.

continuum and its services (U.S. House of Representatives, 1980). At the left side of the continuum are those services that do not place any restrictions on the behavior of older persons. As services are listed toward the right, they become more restrictive. Nursing homes are a major example of a restrictive service. Nursing homes restrict individual freedom in all areas of life, including where to live, with whom to associate, and when and what to eat. Underlying the continuum of services is a supposed continuum of need. As the older person's needs grow, there should be programs and services that match and meet each need.

A variety of ancillary services, such as transportation, underlie the model. The ancillary services enable an older person to reach and use available services. Although there is no doubt about the importance of the ancillary services, questions can be raised about the portrayal of health services in this model. Compared to the services listed under institutional care, the health care services are perceived as acute/episodic. Health care services needed in effective home health care may address chronic needs and be long-term in nature. More importantly, however, serious problems underlie the concept of the continuum of care.

Viewed in terms of an ideal type, the continuum may be valid, but it does not represent the reality of American programs and services for the aged. The continuum of care model is based on the faulty assumption that an individual has only one need at any one point in time. Older people, as indeed all individuals, have many needs at the same time. The needs of the older person are often extensive and include services such as physical therapy, help in ambulation, alleviation of poor vision or hearing, and relief from pain caused by chronic conditions such as arthritis. A particular program or service may be able to meet one of these needs, but not all. The older individual does not move from needing one program or service to needing another. Instead, a package of services is necessary. The components of this package may vary over time.

The continuum of care and continuum of need are also premised on the belief that the same services can be used to meet the needs of all individuals, regardless of their ethnic backgrounds. Nursing homes are viewed as a viable response to the needs of all seriously impaired elderly. This assumption needs to be carefully scrutinized. If a culture frowns upon institutional placements for older persons, nursing homes may not be an acceptable means of assistance. Alternative models, more attuned to the culture, are examined in this chapter's brief discussion of each service. The discussion follows the continuum, by first examining the least restrictive services, then the most restrictive and less utilized services.

Beyond the basic need for nourishment, food and drink can take on many symbolic meanings, for example, the toasts that are part of many ceremonial occasions. Food is also a central part of most social gatherings. The social aspects of eating may be a factor in the negative attitudes toward eating expressed by many people who live alone. It is therefore not surprising that the first major effort of the OAA was the congregate meals program.

Congregate Meals

Congregate meals are currently the most widely utilized programs funded through the OAA. In 1999, over 113 million meals were served to 1.8 million individuals over the age of 60, at congregate meal sites (Older American Reports, 2002). The congregate meals programs attempt to alleviate two major problems that can affect the older person: the inability to purchase nutritious meals, and the inability to prepare nutritious meals. By offering a properly balanced meal at no cost, congregate meals programs attempt to prevent the onset of malnutrition and illnesses related to malnutrition. There is also the possibility of involving meals programs attendees in a variety of supportive services, including health promotion and general socializing. These supportive services have become a very important element of many congregate nutrition sites.

Ethnic Foods

As already noted, food is a very important part of ethnic identity, and it may become even more important as other characteristics, such as ethnic dress, the mother tongue, and the ethnic neighborhood, become less common. Nutrition programs are often criticized for their failure to provide not only balanced meals, but meals that are representative of the ethnic culture. This criticism should not be accepted without further examination.

As is true of all programs and services, congregate meals programs have the potential to bridge some of the differences among ethnic elderly, or to maintain their solidarity and sense of identity. It is difficult to accomplish both of these goals concurrently. The serving of ethnic foods can provide a sense of order and continuity to older persons from specific ethnic backgrounds. This continuity may be most important for those older individuals who have left their home country at a later age. Such groups would include older Russian Jews who arrived in the United States during the 1970s, or older Vietnamese refugees forced to leave Vietnam.

Unfortunately, nutritional requirements and food preferences are not always in accord. In one case, a Baltimore-based Native American group, interested in the establishment of a nutrition site oriented to older Native Americans, approached an urban Area Agency on Aging for funding. The menu presented for the agency's approval did not meet the requirement that all nutrition program lunches provide one third the government-established dietary allowances. The Native Americans argued that it would be impossible to ask older people to change their traditional eating habits. Afraid to violate federal regulations, the Area Agency on Aging responded that they could not authorize the Native American nutrition site.

That the aged prefer to only eat food prepared according to their ethnic traditions may also be an incorrect assumption. An older Nisei (second-generation Japanese American) may enjoy Japanese food, but may also relish standard American fare. The same enjoyment of diverse food may be true of fourth-generation Mexican Americans or third-generation Jewish Americans.

Meals on Wheels

Meals on Wheels programs are now found in most developed countries. The target population is older people who are not ambulatory, cannot prepare their own meals, and cannot leave their homes to attend a congregate nutrition program. Volunteers bring the meals to the older person's home and check on their basic condition. In 1999, 135 million home-delivered meals were provided to 883,000 clients throughout the United States (Older American Reports, 2002).

The Meals on Wheels volunteer may be the only social contact some older people have during the week. An effort to match the ethnic backgrounds of volunteers with those of recipients can break through the isolation of homebound older persons. Matching is most likely to be possible in communities with a concentration of older persons from a particular ethnic background.

Care must be taken if this matching effort is to be effective. Data sheets must not only ascertain whether volunteers or recipients are African American, White, Latino, Asian, or Native American, but it is important to distinguish, for example, between older Haitians and older African Americans. In the same manner, the category "Asian" fails to reveal enough information about the ethnic background of an individual to promote optimal matching of volunteers and recipients. Among older Vietnamese, inquiring whether the older person is from a Chinese background is important, because there have always been substantial numbers of Chinese living in Vietnam. In the same manner, Italian or Jewish communities might be served by matched volunteers, if the agency is careful to obtain information on ethnic background. Attention to the quality of the delivered meals should not be forgotten. To an older person from an ethnic community whose food has a particular style of preparation and seasoning, mass-produced meals available through Meals on Wheels may seem bland, uninteresting, and unenticing. Although delivered with the best intentions, these meals may go uneaten. The quality of the food may be more important to an older person who is homebound than to an older person chatting with others at a congregate nutrition program.

SENIOR CENTERS

After 50 years of growth, what exactly comprises a senior center remains unclear. Directories of senior centers include organizations and programs that often are widely disparate in their extensiveness, as well as orientation. Ralston (1987) notes five major definitions of senior centers. All of the definitions are broad-based in their specification of programmatic elements. An alternative to the varied definitions is adoption of a model that stresses core services: These help to distinguish between senior centers and nutrition sites, which serve meals and have few additional services. The core services recommended in one study (Gelfand, Bechill, & Chester, 1991) include:

- Congregate meals
- Home-delivered meals
- Exercise
- Information and assistance
- Socializing
- Transportation

There are differentials in the health, mental health, and living conditions that create problems for older persons from various ethnic groups, but the above list of core services appears to fit the basic needs of all groups. The manner in which some of these services are offered differs according to the needs and cultural norms of the specific group of ethnic aged.

Exercise Programs

The configuring of meals programs to meet the needs and desires of ethnic aged is discussed above. Exercise programs will differ according to the respective health conditions of the older ethnic aged. There are, however, issues related to the conduct of these programs.

Some cultures segregate activities of men and women and place restrictions on "immodesty" in dress. Programs that serve Arab Americans who are Muslims need to consider Islamic norms about appropriate activities and dress for women. Women from other cultures may also regard exercises as demeaning and unbefitting an older woman's status.

Information and Assistance

Information and assistance are crucial aspects of programs for the aged in all communities, and are offered by a variety of providers. Information and assistance are based on the assumption that the older person, or an individual in contact with the older person, recognizes a need and makes an effort to obtain aid. As already discussed, this assumption may not be valid and may create problems in conducting effective outreach efforts. In some situations, in which the prevalence of a health or functional problem is high, the older person may regard it as either normal or impossible to modify.

The adaptation of the affected individuals and their community to problematic behavior may be accepted as normal, even if this adaptation impairs the functioning of the older person. An example of this process is the acceptance of alcohol abuse as normal behavior. Equally problematic is the unwillingness of older people to acknowledge alcohol abuse. If it is recognized as undesirable behavior, the stigma attached to alcohol abuse may prevent many older persons or their families from admitting their need and seeking assistance.

Behaviors that result from certain diseases associated with aging, particularly Alzheimer's, also retard acceptance of the need for help.

This is clarified in a description of the response of one Latino family to the behavior of an Alzheimer's patient:

> Even during a time when her husband was so confused that he was urinating on the living room floor, Mrs. Garcia tried to put up a front that everything was okay to her neighbors certainly but also even to her children. (Henderson, Alexander, & Gutierrez-Mayka, n.d., p. 17)

After Mrs. Garcia's husband wandered away, he was found by a neighbor about two miles from home. "His safety as well as the public nature of his 'crazy behavior' mortified Mrs. Garcia" (p. 18), who viewed the symptoms of Alzheimer's as those of a very stigmatized mental illness that would also stigmatize the family.

Seeking assistance for the older person from formal providers can be viewed as a reduction in the importance of the informal social network within the ethnic group. To older people and their adult children, initiating formal service delivery may represent an abdication of responsibility or failure on their part to provide the assistance that is expected from them.

As one Vietnamese refugee commented about family responsibilities: "The family is a hospital. If mom is sick, my children and my brother and my sisters care for her. We don't need a nurse. She stays home, so we don't need to send her to a nursing home" (Gold, 1992).

The demands of urban America make it difficult for many Vietnamese families to fulfill their perceived obligations to their parents, yet they may delay inquiries about available services. Variations in ethnic norms, about the role of family in caregiving, mandate special sensitivity among staff involved in information and assistance programs. A major, usually reluctant, shift in attitude is often required before Vietnamese families inquire about formal services for their older relatives. In answering these requests, any implication that the family has failed to shoulder appropriate responsibilities should be avoided. Staff also need to stress how the provision of services will support, rather than substitute for, the family's assistance efforts.

Socializing

Socializing is an important senior center function that is often overlooked. For Soviet Jews who are concerned about the isolation of their parents, the opportunities for socializing offered by a senior center may be its most important activity. There are, however, both ethnic and age cohort issues in socializing. As already noted, some groups will not feel comfortable socializing with individuals from other backgrounds. Physical space or separate time allocations must be utilized to allow disparate or historically antagonistic groups to meet. Older men may also want to have the opportunity to socialize without the presence of women, and the same may be true for older women. These preferences may reflect ethnic culture, but may be less true among younger age cohorts, who are more accustomed to sexually integrated and less gender-specific activities. Men and women in their sixties may also not want to attend a center where the clientele is predominantly in their late seventies and eighties.

Transportation

On the surface, it is difficult to envision differences in transportation related to ethnic background. Obviously, ethnic differences cannot account for different forms of transportation being offered by an agency. To some degree, usage patterns may be explainable in terms of place of origin of particular ethnic groups. Older people from rural areas may find mass transit confusing and frightening. The fear may be heightened by the close contact with other people, particularly people from other backgrounds. Combined with a limited ability to read signs and ask directions, ethnic elderly from a rural area may feel more comfortable in cars that take them directly to their destination. As in socializing programs, men and women from particular ethnic backgrounds may not feel comfortable sitting near each other in subways or buses, or even in vans utilized for transportation to programs.

Supplementary Senior Center Services

Beyond the basic list, there are a number of supplementary programs that senior centers may find worthwhile to provide. The supplementary programs and services offered by a center for the ethnic elderly may relate as much to cohort issues as needs. Classes in English may be useful for recent immigrants negotiating the American service-delivery system. Facility in English also makes it possible for Latino or Asian elderly to shop, use public transportation, or develop friendships among individuals outside their own ethnic group. Language classes may also be welcomed by second- and third-generation ethnic aged who have limited or no ability in their mother tongue, but who see the language as a link to their ethnic background. The mother tongue plays this role for many Estonians, who use Estonian at church and at summer camp settings (Walko, 1989).

Senior center services can be planned on the assumption that individuals from a particular ethnic background may lack knowledge of other cultures, or even their own. This is particularly true of older individuals whose interest in their ethnic background has only revived. Their interests may extend to learning about the traditional elements of the culture, which could include history, rituals, and native crafts.

The revival of ethnic crafts can be a major factor in the development of greater self-esteem among members of the group, as demonstrated by the strong interest shown in traditional Pueblo pottery. This craft form was rapidly disappearing until a few Pueblo artists, particularly Maria Martinez of the San Ildefonso pueblo, rediscovered traditional black pottery and began to teach the traditional methods to younger individuals. Older Soviet Jews may show a strong interest in Jewish culture, because of their inability to participate in any religious observance while living in the Soviet Union. Dance and music programs related to ethnic culture may also garner an enthusiastic response among many ethnic elderly.

Ethnic differences, rather than similarities, can be used as a valuable program tool. Programming that brings together various ethnic groups to discuss ethnic differences may foster intragroup cohesion, as well as intergroup understanding. A senior center in Rhode Island sponsors an ethnic day focused around the Easter holidays. At this ethnic day, participants from different ethnic groups discuss how they celebrate Easter. Similarities are sometimes the basis for extensive discussions, but differences allow participants to proudly proclaim the importance and distinctiveness of their holiday celebrations.

A further example is provided by the use of the National Council on Aging humanities programs at a congregate meals site. The humanities series utilized first-person descriptions taken from autobiographies and reports about specific events. One is by a Jewish woman, describing how her family celebrated winter in Russia when she was a child. On the surface, this description has little to do with the lives of the older African American men and women attending a congregate meals program in Indianapolis, but, used at this site, the description sparked substantial discussion. These men and women found similarities, as well as differences, between their own lives and the events of the Jewish ghettos of Russia. The discussion was both interesting and insightful.

The inception of ethnically oriented programming must be done carefully, in order to avoid charges that the center is catering only to one ethnic group. This has happened in Australia, where centers are funded by local governments, but no provision is made for staff salaries. In these situations, local volunteers administer the centers, and one ethnic group may become dominant. Other ethnic groups avoid the centers, because they feel unwelcome. This situation is less likely to happen in the United States, where centers can be expected to at least have a paid director, even if they are part-time. The director's role is to learn the needs of various groups of ethnic aged and to meet these needs without developing an "in-group" atmosphere.

ADULT DAY CARE CENTERS

Adult day care programs are a growing element in the service armament for impaired older people and are basically targeted to frail elderly. In 1997, there were an estimated 4,000 adult day care centers in operation across the United States (Administration on Aging, 2001a). Operated on a scheduled, rather than a drop-in, basis, the centers provide individualized programs. These individualized efforts are needed, because of the frail health or cognitive problems of the clients. Adult day care clients usually spend two or three days a week at the center. Centers typically have 20–30 older persons in attendance. Many centers provide transportation to and from their facilities.

The physical frailties or cognitive problems of an adult day care client do not necessarily mean that they have lost their individual characteristics. The older person who requires an intensive adult day care program may suffer from severe infirmities. They are still, however, not just older clients, but older African American, older Latino, or older Greek clients, with unique histories and backgrounds. Specific activities, such as crafts, dance programs, or discussions, may be able to utilize the ethnic background of the participants.

For some adult day care participants, attendance has been a reluctant decision, often made under pressure from children or a spouse. Upset about the implication that they need adult day care, the older person may view their participation in the center as an abrogation of traditional caregiving responsibilities by their family. This emotional upset may be directed into anger at family members or into depression. The anger may also be channeled toward individuals from other ethnic or racial groups. Long-standing prejudices may surface in remarks and behavior about other day care participants.

In day care centers where the clients have severe cognitive impairments, short-term memory may be more affected than long-term memory. Long-term memory, including memories of ethnic celebrations, may remain much more intact. These memories can be used in reality therapy and discussions, to assist the older persons' overall functioning. Ethnic objects and related religious objects may spark interest and recognition on the part of cognitively impaired older persons.

EMPLOYMENT PROGRAMS

Employment programs for older persons are funded through Title V of the OAA. This program is available only to lower-income older people. The Title V program is available to individuals whose income is less than 125% of the federal poverty level.

Many of the current cohort of individuals over the age of 55 have limited skills and education that restrict the number of job opportunities available to them. A lack of fluency in English among many ethnic aged also limits the type of positions in which they can be placed or the training that can be provided. In addition, attitudes toward jobs vary culturally. Professionals from India may resent lower-level positions that are located for them through Title V. They may also regard acceptance of these positions as a serious loss of face, a loss that is important in many cultures. For Vietnamese refugees, the shift to a lower job position, necessitated by their move from Vietnam, is also a loss of face. As a Title V job counselor explained,

> For Americans, working is a matter of doing something to survive. For many Asians, the work you do is who you are, and I have been unable to place many older refugees in jobs that they believe were beneath their status, even though they understood that these jobs were the difference between starvation and eating. (Nguyen, personal communication, February 1987)

HOME CARE

Home care has become a major component of the long-term care system, and is usually provided informally by family or friends of the older person. Despite the enormous involvement of family members in assistance to the older person, home care is an increasingly important element in the service-delivery system. Home care can range from nursing services to chore services, such as housekeeping, laundry, and cooking, to personal care, such as assistance with dressing and hairdressing.

All of these services appear to be basic in nature and require the same skills from the provider, regardless of whether the client is Korean,

Jewish, African American, or Italian. The obvious generality of the care needs is deceiving. Many of the home care services require the personal involvement of the caregiver with the recipient. In many cultures, there may be strictures about who is appropriate in these roles and how the services should be provided.

Because of ascribed sex and age roles, Asian men may not be at ease with women from other cultures, especially if these women are younger providers. Latino men may also feel uncomfortable with women as providers of intimate services, such as dressing and bathing. Latino women may also have similar reactions about male providers who violate ethnic norms of modesty.

A focus solely on the technical aspects of the home care provider's work overlooks the importance of the social contact between the older person and the provider. A home care provider has the potential to affect the self-esteem, morale, and sense of control of the older person.

A home care provider from the same ethnic background as the client could have the optimal effect. Shared cultural background and values between the provider and client can be employed in a therapeutic manner with the older client. Achieving this therapeutic effect requires attention to factors other than technical proficiency in the training of in-home workers. As Sheehan's (1984) description of the process of obtaining capable in-home workers indicates, few minimum-wage home care workers are trained to maximize the potential social and therapeutic effects of their presence in an older person's home.

RESIDENTIAL FACILITIES

Many workers in residential facilities come to believe that age is really a leveler. Their perception of this leveling effect is based on the similar physical and cognitive needs of older individuals in the residential environment. As the variety of residential facilities for older persons increase, the diversity of populations who live in these facilities will also increase.

Retirement and Life Care Communities

The variety of residential settings planned or available for older persons has increased dramatically. At one extreme are retirement communities, which offer housing physically designed to meet the needs of older persons, but offer few other amenities. In these homes, the light switches are lower on the wall, and all rooms are on one level. Some arrangements may be included to cover all external care of the home, including mowing, snow removal, and maintenance. Large retirement communities of this nature are now in operation in many states.

During the 1990s, there was enormous growth in what is termed *assisted living*. Assisted living can be defined as a "special combination of housing, personalized supportive services and health care designed to meet the needs—both scheduled and unscheduled—of those who need help with activities of daily living" (Assisted Living Foundation of America, n.d.). Because regulations regarding assisted living facilities vary from state to state, there is little uniformity in their services, which often include meals, housekeeping, transportation, assistance with daily activities, access to health and mental health services, health promotion activities and exercise, laundry, management of medications, and a variety of social and recreational activities (Assisted Living Foundation of America, n.d.).

Continuing care retirement communities, or "life-care" communities, have developed in recent years, as a specific type of assisted living environment. These communities guarantee that the individual can stay in the residence they purchase or rent, regardless of changes in their physical condition, and that they will receive care as necessary. If needed, the resident can move to a nursing home facility in the continuing care community. Because of their high entrance fees, or rents, life-care communities remain oriented to older people with high incomes or substantial assets. Such communities usually offer a variety of recreational activities and limited transportation to community programs.

In these varied communities, ethnically oriented programs may be meaningful to the residents. Clubs focused around ethnically based activities and holiday celebrations can be developed in the life care communities. In retirement communities, builders often provide clubhouses for activities and volunteer organizations that assist in meeting transportation needs and the provision of medical equipment. The clubhouses often become the center of community activities. The clubhouse can provide a base for maintenance or redevelopment of ethnic identity among residents in the retirement community. An ethnically based group may involve older residents who might otherwise become isolated, and help new residents adapt to their environment and develop social relationships.

Nursing Homes

Nursing homes represent the most important, but also the most difficult, environment in which to work against the age-as-a-leveler adage. Nursing home residents do not choose to live in this environment, and, among many ethnic groups, there are strong norms against using nursing homes. In the Dallas-Ft.Worth area, Mexican caregivers expressed mistrust of nursing homes and the quality of care their older family members would receive in these facilities (John & McMillan, 1998). In focus groups and interviews with 60 African Americans, there was a strong feeling that nursing homes were not desirable settings for older persons and should be avoided (Groger, Mayberry, & Straker, 2001). In each of the eight focus groups, however, there was at least one participant who had utilized nursing home placement for a relative. The low use of nursing homes by some ethnic groups may also result from a lack of referrals by providers, who may believe that the group is better able to care for an impaired older person than is actually true (Finn, n.d.).

Older individuals in nursing homes have major physical infirmities or cognitive problems that prevent them from living in any other alternative setting. As community care options become more extensive, a greater proportion of nursing homes are becoming skilled nursing facilities, where the major tasks of the day are what have been described as "bed and body" work. These tasks include waking the resident, monitoring the resident's dressing and preparation for mealtimes, and cleaning the room. Similar tasks are required during the day and before bedtime. For seriously impaired residents, the tasks of the nursing home aide may include dressing and bathing the resident, and assistance with toileting and feeding.

Considering ethnic factors in carrying out these basic tasks is difficult for aides and nurses. However, there are differences among ethnic groups in the ways in which they expect to be addressed. The older person may view violation of these rules of etiquette as a deliberate insult. These perceived insults may be intensified if nursing home staff does not respect the privacy of the older person, particularly their modesty about dressing, toileting, and bathing.

The ethnic background of the resident can also be carefully utilized in nursing homes as a therapeutic element. Even if their short-term memory is cognitively impaired, nursing home residents may still feel more comfortable living in the company of residents from the same cultural background. Since long-term memory is often unimpaired in individuals, the sharing of past experiences can help nursing home residents develop a sense of commonality and friendship.

Some ethnic groups are large enough and have enough economic resources to develop nursing homes that cater primarily to the group. In most cases, however, it can be expected that there will be a mixture of ethnic groups in a nursing home. In communities with large numbers of Greeks, Italians, or Latinos, a clustering approach may be possible. Clustering involves grouping individuals from the same ethnic background together in rooms or in wings of a nursing home. Once this clustering is accomplished, a variety of ethnically oriented programs can be planned that may help to develop social relationships among residents.

HEALTH PROGRAMS AND ETHNICITY

The overwhelming share of public funds devoted to health care for older people is spent on two reimbursement mechanisms, Medicare and Medicaid, which ensure that older people are not denied access to health care because of costs. By themselves, they do not create new programs and services. The important issues related to ethnic background and health services can best be examined by a division of health care into primary prevention and secondary prevention.

Primary Prevention

Primary prevention attempts to deter the onset of illness. As more knowledge is gained, it is evident that chronic, as well as acute, health conditions can be prevented through an individual's behavior when they are young. One example is the onset of osteoporosis among older women. Many cases of osteoporosis could be prevented by an increased intake of calcium and more exercise among women—even young women. Other prevention programs stress balanced diet, limits on alcohol and drug use, and cessation of smoking. Even if individuals have not had good health habits in earlier years, significant improvements in health can still take place with changes in lifestyle when people are older. Recent studies demonstrate the benefits of exercise for older people, including weight-based exercises. Smoking cessation results in better lung conditions and breathing among people of all ages.

Among ethnic elderly with limited educational backgrounds, there may be a lack of knowledge about proper nutrition and smoking. Low incomes also force many ethnic elderly to adopt a diet that does not include balanced meals. Programs that provide ethnic elderly with information about primary prevention in health care are important, but not necessarily sufficient, to produce a change in lifestyles.

Health programs initiated with the ethnic aged must take into account different health belief systems. An example can be seen in Vietnamese culture, in which there are three explanations for illness (Tung, 1980). The first is that illness is caused by a natural phenomenon, such as spoiled food. This explanation promotes the use of herbs and diets to solve health problems. In the Vietnamese community, knowledge about herbal remedies has been passed on intergenerationally. In the second explanation, illnesses are caused by supernatural powers, such as gods, demons, and spirits. In these cases, the disease may be a punishment, or may be brought on by the malevolence of other individuals. The third explanation is based on the hot or cold theory and is common to Vietnam, Japan, and Korea. According to this theory, the body operates in a balance between Yin and Yang. Excesses in either direction lead to illness. An excess of cold elements may produce diarrhea, but an excess of hot elements produces pimples. The principles of hot and cold are carried over into treatment, in order to restore a balance between these elements. In the case of the common cold, fluid intake is restricted, because it brings more cold elements into the body, which is already out of balance.

Among Mexican Americans, *curanderisimo* represents a long-standing belief system. These beliefs explain the onset and causes of misfortunes and illness. Five major elements can be found in this belief system:

1. the ancient humoral theory of illness
2. characterological strengths and weaknesses that relate to individual susceptibility to illness
3. "naturalistic" folk conditions, such as *Caida de mollera* (collapsed fontanel in infants) and *empacho* (intestinal distress)
4. mystical cases, such as fate, destiny, *susto* (soul loss), and *mal ojo* (evil eye)
5. magical causes, such as *embrujo* (witchcraft) and *mal puesto* (hexing) (Ness & Wintrob, 1981, p. 1479)

Among Puerto Ricans, *espiritismo* is a system of beliefs that incorporates elements from Spanish, African, and Indian healing practices. Esperitismo is based on the "belief that the visible and invisible worlds are inhabited by spirits that are temporarily encased in a human body in the material world" (Ness & Wintrob, 1981, p. 1479). At times, these spirits have difficulty achieving their mission and intrude on people's bodies. This intrusion causes both physical and psychological distress.

One group of researchers has explored the attitudes of African Americans, Latinos, and Filipinos concerning chronic illness. The research participants were between the ages of 49 and 97 (Becker, Beyne, Newsom, & Rodgers, 1998). The beliefs of the African Americans were consistent with mainstream U.S. medical beliefs. Filipino Americans also had views that were consistent with American attitudes about health, and they recognized the value of a number of health practices. Carrying out these practices and maintaining good health extended beyond concerns for their own well-being and also was viewed as part of their responsibility to the family.

The Latino views of health were a contrast. The 61 Latino men and women had limited knowledge about health conditions and their possible role in the management of chronic illnesses. The limited knowledge included not understanding possible causes of their illness. If the symptoms of a chronic illness disappeared when they took medication, they believed they were cured of the illness. Each new episode of the illness was viewed as a sign of a separate illness. Prescription drugs were solely relied upon to control their illness.

The data from this type of research indicates that primary prevention, for the ethnic aged, must first be based on an evaluation of the positive and negative impacts of the indigenous belief systems on the health of the older person. Second, a careful assessment is needed to ascertain whether these long-standing beliefs have developed because of a lack of availability or knowledge of alternative health care models. If the beliefs are strongly embedded in cultural values, an attempt to convince the older person that these belief systems are unfounded is likely to fail.

The problems that can result when traditional ethnic health practices are discarded, regardless of their impact, is illustrated by dietary changes. The diets of some ethnic aged have changed over the years, as they have become acculturated to American lifestyles. Rather than stir-fried vegetables, they may have adopted diets with a high meat and fat content. The negative impact of these changes can be seen in the higher incidence of some illnesses among American-born Chinese than in their peers born in mainland China. It is impossible to assert that these figures are totally related to diet, but diet has been earmarked as one major component in morbidity and mortality statistics. Primary prevention for the ethnic aged must include helping the older person maintain the traditional health beliefs that are positive, while incorporating new health care practices that will be beneficial.

Secondary Prevention

Secondary prevention is an effort to reduce the duration of an illness. Early detection and treatment of an illness can reduce its duration. This statement is more true about acute than chronic conditions. Effective secondary prevention programs can, however, prevent worsening of the chronic condition. These secondary prevention efforts bring individuals into early contact with the health care system. Clinics and community outreach programs that involve the older person in health screening may alert practitioners to health conditions before these conditions impair the older person's functioning. Effective secondary prevention must therefore deal with issues of service availability and accessibility.

With the ethnic aged, there is also the additional question of understanding symptoms as described and related by an older person. Nurses and physicians may not understand a Vietnamese patient's meaning when he talks about being hot, but seems to have no fever. Possibly, over time, Southeast Asians will begin to incorporate a more Western approach to health care. This does not necessarily imply extinction of the culture's approach to illness prevention and treatment. More likely, it will be a merger of the two approaches. Traditional medicine and Western medicines will be used in combination for some illnesses. This type of syncretism can be seen in the interest in acupuncture in the United States. Adherents of this traditional Chinese treatment modality see no conflict between its usage and the Western emphasis on medication. Older Chinese in Boston use both Western and Chinese medicine. Chinese medicine is viewed as appropriate for minor and chronic disorders. Western medicine is relied upon for treatment of major and acute health problems (Liu, 1986).

For Latinos, *curanderos* and *espiritistas* represent important community-based health care providers. The practices of *curanderos* can be described as fitting into a model of holistic medicine. A variety of diets, herbs, rituals, and massages, as well as prayer, are employed by *curanderos*. There are also important folk-healing systems that are indigenous to Native American tribes, which employ prayer, rituals, diets, and, in some cases, sweat baths.

Many providers may regard these Chinese, Latino, and Native American beliefs, about the causes and treatment of illness, as unscientific and unworthy of consideration in treatment. This attitude can produce major tensions between the health care, provider and the ethnic older person. The older Vietnamese person may disregard prescriptions about health care, because they do not correspond with indigenous beliefs. The older Dominican may believe that "God guides one's destiny," that their illness is a result of "God's will" (Paulino, 1998, p. 69) and that the doctor's advice is useless in confronting their illness. In these cases, the health care provider's treatment plan may be ignored. Perhaps more dangerous is the combination of indigenous health practices with prescribed medical treatments. The use of herbal and folk remedies may mitigate the effects of prescription drugs. These herbal remedies may also increase the effects of prescription drugs or produce drug interactions.

The development of an effective secondary prevention model for the ethnic aged necessitates some knowledge of the indigenous health care system on the part of health care providers. This knowledge must include not only an understanding of what a patient means when describing a symptom, but also an ability to assess whether indigenous remedies, such as herbs, are being used in treatment and what these remedies are. It is important, however, not to overgeneralize about the allegiance of people to culturally based health beliefs or health providers. Older Latinos may have more allegiance to these forms of folk healing than younger Mexican Americans or Puerto Ricans. Even among older Mexican Americans, adherence to traditional indigenous healers may vary between United States- and Mexican-born older persons. In a major national survey of all age groups, undertaken between 1982 and 1984, only 4% of Mexican Americans had consulted *curanderos* during the past 12 months (Higgenbotham, Trevino, & Ray, 1990).

With the revival of knowledge and interest in their culture among Native Americans, extensive use of native healers has been found, for example, among Navajos (Kim & Kwok, 1998), Native American patients in an urban clinic in Wisconsin (Marbella, Harris, Diehr, Ignace, & Ignace, 1998), and Native Americans patients interviewed in the Seattle area (Buchwald, Beals, & Manson, 2000).

An obvious requirement of health programs for older persons is cultural competence among the providers. Understanding of an ethnic culture, however, is not sufficient. The programs that are developed also need to take cultural beliefs into account. Bringing native healers or respected community leaders into the education and treatment process may help to bridge the gap between the formal health care system and the ethnic community.

One example is the Collaborative Health Education Training Program (Administration on Aging, 2001b), which was an effort targeted to increasing the understanding of African American ministers and community agency staff about health care problems in the Black community. The program included 56 hours of "train the trainer" sessions on a variety of health issues, ranging from diabetes to heart disease. After the training, the ministers and community agency staff then trained individuals in their own communities. Networking among the different community agencies and ministers increased as a result of the program's efforts.

End-of-Life Services

Although interdisciplinary in nature, end-of-life services are predominantly health-oriented services that also provide emotional and instrumental support to a terminally ill individual and their family. Hospice programs are the most widely known end-of-life service, but, in recent years, the field has been attempting to broaden its purview to palliative care, which may or may not be linked to hospice efforts.

In the United States, the majority of hospice patients are older individuals with cancer. In order to qualify for Medicare reimbursement for hospice care, the individual must have a prognosis of no more than 6 months of life remaining. The majority of hospice care is provided at home and includes pain management, counseling with families, religious support, and provision of needed equipment, such as hospital beds. Palliative care also stresses pain management and comfort, but may be provided to individuals who are not terminally ill.

There is still only limited knowledge about the role of ethnicity in attitudes about end-of-life, palliative care, and hospice, and only a small proportion of hospice clients are from a minority status. Part of this limited use of palliative care may stem from a lack of knowledge, or misunderstanding, of palliative care. It may also stem from a concern that palliative care may attempt to displace the family in its efforts to provide care for the terminally ill individual. Research with Mexicans in Michigan and Arizona indicated a willingness to utilize palliative care, but also a desire for hospice providers to limit their role to a strictly medical function (Gelfand, Balcazar, Parzuchowski, & Lenox, 2001).

Similarities and differences have been found in end-of-life attitudes among Asians. One of the similarities is a valuing of longevity over quality of life and a belief that patients should not be told about any terminal illness (Yeo & Hikoyeda, 2000). These beliefs limit the willingness of many Asian groups to make extensive use of hospice programs. Among African Americans, the mistrust of the health care system may also extend to hospice programs that are viewed as part of the health care system. The attitudes that now restrict the use of palliative care by many ethnic groups may change among upcoming generations of ethnic aged. Hopefully, these older people will have had better experiences with the American health care system, or a change in their beliefs as a result of acculturation.

MENTAL HEALTH SERVICES AND ETHNICITY

Mental Health Services Availability

Since the 1970s, mental health treatment has shifted from inpatient units at state mental hospitals to outpatient services in the community. In 1970, the census of state hospital patients was a rate of 186 per 100,000 individuals. By 1992, this rate had dropped to 33 per 100,000 individuals. In the past, older patients were a large part of the inpatient population of mental hospitals, but a small part of outpatient clinics. Hospitals contained older patients who had entered many years before and aged in the hospital. Although mental health clinics have a long history in the United States, community-based mental health services have multiplied extensively since the 1960s. The Community Mental Health Act of 1963 fostered the development of community mental health centers throughout the country. Placed in so-called "catchment areas" of approximately 175,000 residents, these centers were designed to serve the specific needs of the population in the area.

By the mid-1970s, there were extensive community complaints about the centers' lack of attention to the ethnic characteristics of the residents. As a result of these complaints, amendments to the Community Mental Health Act in 1975 required that federally funded mental health centers provide care that "overcomes the geographic, linguistic and economic barriers to the receipt of services" (U.S. Senate, 1975, p. 47), and that centers develop a full range of diagnostic and treatment services for older adults. This mandate should have expanded the attention paid to the special mental health needs of the ethnic aged.

In 1981, funding of federal mental health programs shifted to a block grant approach, in which states were awarded funds, based on the size of the population. The block grants also gave states control over programmatic decisions. By the mid-1980s, state and local governments had managed to keep mental health programs operational at levels comparable to those before the block grant system was instituted. Left to their own decision-making, however, states and localities drew back from an extensive involvement in mental health services for the aged. Lebowitz (1987) cites major factors that have prevented adequate outpatient mental health services from being available to older persons in the community. Included are reimbursement problems, the lack of mental health professionals trained to work with older people, the lack of outreach to older people, and stereotypes about mental illness on the part of both mental health professionals and older people. Professionals have tended to view older persons as uninterested in mental health treatment and as untreatable. Cost and accessibility also inhibit the use of community-based mental health services by the ethnic aged.

Individuals with mental health problems can function well in the community, if they are provided the range of support services they need (Manderscheid & Henderson, 2000). As the number of patients in state hospitals have declined, the responsibility for mental health services has shifted to a variety of local community agencies. It is not clear, however, that many of these communities have the funding needed to provide the gamut of mental health services needed in the community.

The negative attitudes of professionals regarding mental health treatment of adult persons, and the funding problems facing community-based programs, are both factors in the lack of mental health options for African American and other community-based elderly.

Mental Health Service Usage

Attitudes toward mental health among ethnic groups are complex. In many senses, *curanderos* are involved as much with the individual's mental health as their physical health. Some ethnic cultures, including Latinos and Asians, do not separate the health and mental health aspects of an illness. Somatization of a mental health problem is often encountered among Latinos, who may consult spiritualists about problems that include mental health as well as physical health concerns. Asians have also been found to detail their physical complaints to a health care provider without mentioning their emotional problems (U.S. Surgeon General, 2001). The spiritual aspects of these problems are viewed as outside the control of the individual. In many cases, *espiritistas* are able to exorcise these negative spirits. If the *espiritista* is unable to meet the needs of the individual, it is important that they refer their clients to other mental health providers. But these referrals may never take place, because these indigenous providers are not linked to the formal mental health system. Many ethnic populations also utilize other alternatives before seeking professional help. In Tennessee, African American elderly, suffering from upset, worry, nerves, or emotional problems, primarily alleviate these problems by themselves (92%), frequent prayer (92%), talking to friends/relatives (74%), talking to spouse/family

(67%), or listening to music (36%). If formal assistance is sought, clergy and family doctors are the most likely source. Clergymen are used more as a source of assistance by women than by men (Husaini, Moore, & Cain, 1991).

The NSBA indicated that, of those older African Americans who sought professional help for a mental health problem, 18% went to a hospital, 17% to a doctor, 7% to a minister, and 4% to a social service agency. The percentage of African American elderly seeking professional help of any kind declined with age, from 53% among individuals ages 55–64, to 33% among individuals over age 75 (Greene, Jackson, & Neighbors, 1993). Similarly, the percentage of African American elderly who used informal help also declined with age, from 85% among those aged 55–64, to 53% among those over age 75. The large number of African American elderly over age 75, who are "nonusers" of any type of help, is an indication of substantial unmet mental health needs among this group of elderly. Overall, 58% of older African Americans do not receive needed mental health treatment (U.S. Surgeon General, 2001).

Ethnicity and Mental Health Treatment

The ethnic aged person can place new demands on the mental health worker. If the worker does not speak the language of the older person, a translator may have to be employed, which places a barrier between the worker and client. A translator may unintentionally alter the meaning of what the client is trying to communicate. Any translation requires modifications, since words that have meaning in one language cannot always be translated exactly into another language.

Besides the problems in meaning introduced by translations, the client may feel constrained about speaking in front of a translator. This may be particularly true if the translator is from the same ethnic background and lives in the same community as the client. In these cases, the translator may intentionally alter the client's words if they feel that what the client is saying reflects badly on the ethnic community.

Negative professional attitudes about treating older people are often matched among older people who have negative attitudes about mental health problems. Many older persons view mental health problems as signs of personal failure or spiritual deficiency (Lebowitz, 1987).

For many ethnic aged, mental health services also carry the stigma of "craziness." As one Vietnamese social worker commented:

> I think the difficulty is that there is a lack of understanding of mental health as it is understood in this country. For an average Vietnamese, mental health would immediately mean that the person is crazy, acting crazy, saying crazy things. But to us, a mental health problem could also be that the person is experiencing marital problems, a person is having difficulty in dealing with a coworker, for an adolescent having difficulty establishing or maintaining peer relationships, you know, to have friends. These are the kinds of problems that we would work with. (Gold, 1992, p. 152)

In addition to the fact that Vietnamese often do not differentiate between psychological and physical problems, there are three other important elements in the way Southeast Asians deal with mental health (Lin & Masuda, 1983):

1. Mental health problems are viewed as related to negative life events, such as war or loss of a business.
2. Since families are the basic unit of the society, mental health problems are viewed as a threat to the family equilibrium.
3. Individuals with mental health problems will often seek treatments from providers from different backgrounds and orientations, and disregard the possible contradictions between the various treatments.

If mental health problems are stigmatized by the ethnic culture, consideration should be given to other techniques for introducing mental health issues to ethnic aged. Mental health problems may surface in meetings of older persons who are surrogate parents for their grandchildren, or older persons who are primary caregivers for a spouse. These older persons may exhibit symptoms of stress or depression. Techniques for reducing stress and combating depression can be introduced without reference to mental health problems. The techniques can be included in discussions of how to be an effective caregiver. For older people attempting to deal with functional disabilities, treatment for mental health symptoms can be combined with physical rehabilitation. Combining these two treatments has been shown to significantly reduce the length of hospital stays of impaired patients (Strain et al., 1991).

Mental health problems sometimes underlie the physical health problems of the ethnic aged. Alternatively, mental health problems, particularly depression or paranoia, may result from a decline in health status. A practitioner sensitive to symptoms of mental health problems among diverse ethnic groups will be better able to ensure that treatment for these problems is not ignored. The development of programs and services, sensitive to both the needs and desires of the ethnic aged, is complex. The needs may be attainable, but the desires of the ethnic aged for services may extend beyond the capabilities of most provider organizations and staff. In any case, the services desired by ethnic groups deserve careful consideration.

REFERENCES

Administration on Aging. (2001a). *Final fiscal year 2001 GPRA annual performance plan.* Retrieved June 1, 2002, from *http://www.aoa.dhhs.gov/gpra/gpra2001/ gpra01a.html#clients*

Administration on Aging. (2001b). *Older adults and mental health: Issues and opportunities.* Retrieved June 3, 2002, from *http://www.aoa.dhhs.gov/mh/report2001/*

Aleman, S., & Paz, J. (1998). The Yaqui elderly, cultural oppression and resilience. *Journal of Aging and Ethnicity, 1,* 113–127.

Assisted Living Foundation of America. (n.d.). *Definition of assisted living.* Retrieved June 5, 2002, from *http://www.alfa.org/public/articles/details/cfm?id=96*

Becker, G., Beyene, Y., Newsom, E., & Rodgers, D. (1998). Knowledge and care of chronic illness in three ethnic minority groups. *Family Medicine, 30,* 173–178.

Buchwald, D., Beals, J., & Manson, S. (2000). Use of traditional healing among Native Americans in a primary care setting. *Medical Care, 38,* 1191–1199.

Finn, R. The age-old problem. Retrieved May 14, 2002, from *http://www. research.ucla.edu/chal/html/age_page_shtm*

Gelfand, D., Bechill, W., & Chester, R. (1991). Core programs and services at senior centers. *Journal of Gerontological Social Work, 17,* 145–161.

Gelfand, D., Balcazar, H., Parzuchowski, J., & Lenox, S. (2001). Mexicans and care for the terminally ill: Family hospice and the church. *American Journal of Hospice and Palliative Care, 18,* 391–396.

Gold, S. (1992). *Refugee communities: A comparative field study.* Newbury Park, CA: Sage.

Greene, R., Jackson, J., & Neighbors, H. (1993). Mental health and health seeking behavior. In J. Jackson, L. Chatters, & R. Taylor (Eds.), *Aging in Black America* (pp. 185–202). Newbury Park, CA: Sage.

Groger, L., Mayberry, P., & Straker, J. (2001). *A last resort: African-American elders' use of nursing homes.* Paper presented at the annual meeting of the Gerontological Society of America, Chicago.

Henderson, J., Alexander, L., & Gutierrez-Mayka, M. (n.d). *Minority Alzheimer's caregivers: Removing barriers to community services. A training manual.* Tampa, FL: University of South Florida.

Higgenbotham, J., Trevino, F., & Ray, L. (1990). Utilization of curanderos by Mexican Americans: Prevalence and predictors. Findings from HHANES, 1982–1984. *American Journal of Public Health, 80*(December Suppl.), 32–35.

Husaini, B., Moore, S., & Cain, V. (1991). *Psychiatric symptoms and help-seeking behavior among the elderly: Black-White comparisons.* Paper presented at the annual meeting of the Historic Black Colleges and Universities Gerontological Association, Norfolk, VA.

John, R., & McMillan, B. (1998). Exploring caregiver burden among Mexican Americans: Cultural, prescriptions, family dilemmas. *Journal of Aging and Ethnicity, 1,* 93–112.

Kim, C., & Kwok, Y. (1998). Navajo use of native healers. *Archives of Internal Medicine, 158,* 2245–2249.

Lebowitz, B. (1987). Mental health services. In G. Maddox (Ed.), *The encyclopedia of aging* (pp. 440–442). New York: Springer Publishing.

Lin, K., & Masuda, M. (1983). Impact of the refugee experience: Mental health issues of Southeast Asian refugees. In *Bridging Cultures: Southeast Asian refugees in America* (pp. 32–54). Los Angeles: Asian American Community Mental Health Training Center, Special Services for Groups.

Liu, W. (1986). Health services for Asian elderly. *Research on Aging, 8,* 156–175.

Manderscheid, R., & Henderson, Eds. (2000). *Mental health, United States, 2000.* U.S. Department of Health and Human Services, Substance Abuse and Mental Health Administration. Retrieved June 3, 2002, from *http://www.mentalhealth.org/publications/allpubs/SMA01-3537/default.asp*

Marbella, A., Harrison, M., Diehr, S., Ignace, G., & Ignace, G. (1998). Use of Native American healers among Native American patients in an urban Native American health center. *Archives of Family Medicine, 7,* 182–185.

Markides, K., Liang, J., & Jackson, J. (1990). Race, ethnicity and aging. In R. Binstock & L. George (Eds.), *Handbook of aging and the social sciences* (3rd. ed.) (pp. 112–125). San Diego, CA: Academic Press.

Ness, R., & Wintrob, R. (1981). Folk healing: A description and synthesis. *American Journal of Psychiatry, 138,* 1477–1481.

Older American Reports (2002, March 22). *Special report: 1999 Older Americans Act data.* Bethesda, MD: Author.

Paulino, A. (1998). Dominican immigrant elders: Social service needs, utilization patterns and challenges. *Journal of Gerontological Social Work, 30*(1/2), 61–74.

Ralston, P. (1987). Senior center research: Policy from knowledge? In D. Borgatta & R. Montgomery (Eds.), *Critical issues in aging policy* (pp. 199–234). Newbury Park, CA: Sage.

Sheehan, S. (1984). *Kate Quinton's days.* New York: Houghton Mifflin.

Strain, J., Lyons, J. S., Hammer, J. S., Fahs, M., et al. (1991). Cost offset from a psychiatric consultation-liaison intervention with elderly hip fracture patients. *American Journal of Psychiatry, 148,* 1044–1049.

Tung, T. (1980). *Indochinese patients.* Falls Church, VA: Action for South East Asians.

U.S. House of Representatives. (1980). *Future directions for aging policy: A human service model.* A report by the Subcommittee on Human Services of the Select Committee on Aging. Washington, DC: U.S. Government Printing Office.

U.S. Senate. (1975). *Community mental health centers amendments of 1975* (S.66). Washington, DC: U.S. Government Printing Office.

U.S. Surgeon General. (2001). *Mental health: Culture, race and ethnicity.* Retrieved June 2, 2002, from *http://www.mentalhealth/org/cre/toc.asp*

Walko, M. A. (1989). *Rejecting the second generation hypothesis: Maintaining Estonian identity in Lakewood, New Jersey.* New York: AMS Press.

Yeo, G., & Hikoyeda, N. (2000). Cultural issues in end-of-life decision making among Asians and Pacific Islanders in the United States. In K. Braun (Ed.), *Cultural issues in end-of-life decision making* (pp. 101–126). Thousand Oaks, CA: Sage.

Chapter Eight

Paradigms, Assumptions, and Assessments

The preceding chapters raise many questions for the reader, but leave many of these questions unanswered. The questions are a good indication of how many gaps there are in knowledge about ethnicity and aging. Continued and expanded research is needed. It is doubtful, however, whether the paradigm under which research about ethnicity and aging has been conducted will prove adequate for this future research.

Kuhn (1962) defined *paradigms*, in his famous book, *The Structure of Scientific Revolutions,* as models "from which spring particular coherent traditions of scientific research" (p. 10). In the natural and physical sciences, these models include Ptolemaic astronomy or Newtonian physics. These models define "normal" science in any period of time, and set the boundaries of accepted scientific research.

ASSUMPTIONS OF ETHNICITY AND AGING

Although not commonly thought about in relation to the field of aging, the model of normal science in gerontology includes certain assumptions about the importance of race and ethnicity. Knowledge about African American, Latino, Asian, Native American, and, to some extent, White ethnic aged, has increased under the current assumptions, which are important, because they set not only the agenda for research, but the agenda for programs and services as well. These assumptions are also the basis for the training of service providers from a variety of professions. At least four assumptions frame the discussion of ethnicity and aging at the present time.

Ethnic/Racial Commonalities

The first assumption is that of ethnic/racial group commonalities. The basis for this assumption is the belief that there are strong commonalities across ethnic cultures. Completely discarding or fully supporting this assumption is impossible. To some extent, evaluation of this assumption is a matter of what level of analysis is used. All older people, regardless of their ethnic background, have basic needs that must be met. There are many varied ways to meet these needs.

African Americans, Latinos, and Whites approach the basic physiological changes that result from aging, and changes in social roles, from different perspectives. There may also be biological differences that affect the physiological aging of African Americans, Whites, Latinos, Asians, and Native Americans. If these differences exist, they may account for some of the disparities in morbidity and mortality rates from certain illnesses, such as the high incidence of prostate cancer among African American men. Some of the intense discussion about the reality of the crossover effect stems from the fact that the longevity of African Americans, after a certain age, seems to indicate important biological differences among racial groups.

Intraracial analyses are even more complicated than differentiation between African Americans and Whites. Intraracial analyses indicate that, despite their common racial background, Haitians and African Americans have strong cultural differences that may affect their aging. The differences among Mexicans, Salvadorans, Cubans, and Puerto Ricans are increasingly evident.

Utilization of the assumption of ethnic/racial commonalities results in an ability to discuss Asians or Latinos as a group, and to deliver services targeted at these large populations, without having to consider any more complexity in the planning process. It allows research to be done that combines groups based on the continent from which their families originated, or on the basis of a common spoken language. Sample sizes are increased, and large-scale databases, comparing groups, can be developed. Unfortunately, scientific validity suffers, and will suffer even more as Salvadorans, Guatemalans, Nicaraguans, and other populations from Central America and South America are added to the population designated as Hispanic or Latino.

The lack of differentiation works both for and against the needs of ethnic aged. More attention will be paid to the needs of small ethnic groups if they are viewed as part of a larger Asian, Latino, or Native American population. In some cases, however, the opposite effect occurs. A prime example is the common public image of Asians as the model minority that has no major problems. This image belies the differences among long-settled Asian groups, such as Japanese Americans, and new groups, such as Vietnamese or Cambodians. Most of the members of these latter two groups left their country with little money and only a limited education. On the other hand, Asian Indians who have immigrated to the United States have had the benefits of substantial education.

Among Latinos, the situation of Cuban Americans is vastly different than that of Salvadorans or Nicaraguans in the United States. More educated, with middle-class incomes, the Cuban immigrants of the 1960s have greater socioeconomic resources than Mexican Americans or Central American populations in this country. Later Cuban immigrants, such as those who left via the port of Mariel in 1981, come from lower socioeconomic backgrounds, both in terms of education and income. Research about Latinos that includes Cubans may thus be skewed and show higher socioeconomic status, and fewer health problems than is true among many of the Latino groups in the United States. Research that focuses only on Cubans is questionable when generalized to many other Latino groups, and may also ignore differences within the Cuban population.

At this point in time, there is little knowledge of the differences between the more studied American Indian populations who live west of the Mississippi, such as Navajos, and their counterparts living east of the river. Some of these differences may be related to the reservation or nonreservation residence of Native Americans. An older Chippewa Indian, living on a reservation in upper Michigan, may have less education and fewer assets than an older Chippewa who has grown up and worked in Detroit. Similar comparisons can be made between older African American men and women who live in the rural South, and African American elderly who live in urban areas.

The assumption of commonality among the aged also pervades the field in general. In an analysis of articles in six major gerontology journals between 1982 and 1987, Nelson and Dannefer (1992) noted:

Empirical data to address the hypothesis of increasing variability with age are quite limited. This review . . . revealed that measures of dispersion are reported in nearly half of the studies surveyed. However, statistics were generally noted in a rather incidental way or else not discussed at all; in none of the studies was the topic of diversity a research question. (p. 22)

The authors conclude that diversity, as well as normative age patterns, needs to be considered.

Socioeconomic Affluence and the Aged

The second assumption is the belief in the socioeconomic affluence of the elderly. This assumption gained credibility in the 1980s and early 1990s. As is true of the other assumptions, it is insufficient to describe the total situation of the older American population. It is particularly inadequate in its ability to describe the situation of minority and ethnic aged.

In the 1960s, when attention began to be directed to urban problems and poverty, the older population was seen as a group in need. The nutrition programs begun in 1972 were a response to data that indicated that many older people were eating inadequate meals and suffering from malnutrition. Living on fixed incomes, older Americans were clearly a major component of the poverty population of the United States. Legislation in 1973, which indexed Social Security benefits to the consumer price index, altered the situation for many retirees. Coupled with the increased availability of private pensions for a growing number of employees, the proportion of elderly below the federal poverty index began to decline.

By the 1990s, the percentage of elderly living below the poverty level was less than among other age groups. A common complaint is that too much money is being spent on programs for older people and that children are being shortchanged. Although programs and services for children do require massive additional funding, these continuing complaints fail to recognize the major economic problems among the aged from many ethnic populations. A "misery" index of this type would include many African American, Latino, and Native American aged, as well as some Asian elderly, particularly Southeast Asians. Older people from some European backgrounds also should be included, particularly older widows who are living entirely on low Social Security benefits because their husbands had no pensions and worked in low-paying jobs for most of their lives.

Common Family Orientations

The third assumption stresses the commonalities in family orientations among ethnic groups. Based on the assumptions of commonalities in family orientation, similar programs are planned for many ethnic groups. There are, however, important differences in expectations of family members among the ethnic aged. To some extent, the differences in expectations reflect both traditional cultural norms and responses to conditions that the ethnic group faces. Older Turkish parents prefer to live with their sons. Korean parents also expect to live with their married children. In other cultures, parents expect to live apart from their children for as long as possible, but to receive intensive family assistance as needed.

A corollary of the assumptions of family commonalities is the romantic picture of the family as an institution, in general, and as a provider of assistance to the elderly. The discussion in Chapter 5 indicates that family providers of assistance face many problems and stresses. Conflicts within families are also often overlooked in discussions of the ethnic aged. In some cultures, these conflicts have been incorporated into normative expectations about control of decision-making. In other cultures, the conflicts occur because of norms about appropriate residential arrangements. Although the conflicts may rarely be overtly expressed, they are often just beneath the surface of the formalized relationships in many cultures, and may become apparent when an older person requires assistance from family members. Nydegger (1983) emphasizes that there are few societies in which older people rely solely on their good relationships with family members to obtain assistance when needed. Instead, a variety of control mechanisms are used to garner support, including threats of witchcraft, threats of legal action, rousing of public opinion, or guilt.

Stability of Ethnic Values

The fourth assumption projects a picture of ethnic values as stable and unchanging. Under this assumption, the traditional model is used to guide thinking about the current status of the ethnic group. As argued throughout this book, an alternative is to view ethnicity not only as an ascribed characteristic, but also as having some of the characteristics of an achieved status, that is, characteristics that can be adopted or changed by the individual.

Changes within ethnic groups are sometimes involuntary. A notable example was the shift in power from older to younger persons among Japanese interned in camps in California during World War II. Forced to negotiate with American authorities about details of life in these camps, Japanese-speaking older Issei allowed their Nisei children more of a role in the negotiations than was traditional in Japanese culture.

The shift in authority during this period of Japanese American history permanently altered roles in the Japanese American family (Kitano, 1969).

Transformations in ethnic cultures emerge at different rates among ethnic groups. Age cohort, immigration cohort, and socioeconomic factors all play a vital role in the pace and direction of the change. In the United States, disassociation from being identified with an ethnic group is obviously not possible for racial minorities. There is no guarantee, however, that individuals will not alter their values, even if their visible ethnic characteristics remain the same.

ALTERNATIVE ASSUMPTIONS FOR ETHNICITY AND AGING

Although past assumptions about the ethnic aged may not be relevant to the current diversity in the United States, it is important to formulate alternative assumptions that can be utilized in research, program development, and service delivery. To some degree, these assumptions are the opposite of the existing four discussed above.

Ethnic/Racial Variations

The first alternative assumption is that there are extensive variations among and within ethnic and racial groups, such as African Americans, Latinos, Native Americans, and Asians. Acceptance of this assumption could foster more intensive exploration of the extent to which the ethnic aged differ on a variety of dimensions related to their cultural backgrounds, their history of residence in the United States, and their current social and economic environment.

Socioeconomic Differentiation of the Aged

The second alternative assumption cannot be that of poverty among the elderly, the opposite of assumption number two. Instead, it must be a postulate opposite to Arnold Rose's belief in a developing subculture of the aged discussed in Chapter 1. Where Rose predicted a subculture of the older American population based on increasing numbers of older people from the same socioeconomic background, the truth appears to be that larger numbers of older people produce greater differentiation. Assumption number two must therefore be the assumption of socioeconomic differentiation of the older population.

Family Variability

The third assumption must be that of family variability. Whatever stress may be placed on family values, the family that is now considered to be the traditional model in the United States is no longer the only mode. Differentiation of family forms is occurring among all ethnic groups. Alterations in functions of the family and family roles may accompany changes in family forms. Variability among families has always existed, but has often been overlooked, particularly by Americans interested in assuring themselves that a particular model of family relationships is preferable. Many Americans assert that a nuclear family is the preferred form. However, the 2000 census indicates that less than 25% of all families in the country conform to this model of father and mother with children under the age of 18 (U.S. Census Bureau, 2001).

The assumption of family variability encourages examination of diverse role patterns. These role patterns include the hostile relationships that often exist among families. As Nydegger argues:

> In simple justice it must be pointed out that loving, supportive families can be found in all societies. So can their opposites. We must accept these negative aspects as natural outcomes and attempt to pinpoint those structural features that encourage conflict, before we can fully understand the aged and their family ties. (1983, p. 30)

A family variability assumption also encourages rigorous examination of the validity of the principle of hierarchical compensation in caregiving. As noted in chapter 6, the validity of this principle for Latino families remains a matter of debate. The prevalence among many Native American tribes remains unclear, particularly among tribes that reside on reservations. On the other hand, a hierarchical model may be very operational among Asian Americans, who view the norm of filial piety with great intensity.

Emergent Ethnicity

The fourth assumption is the assumption of emergent ethnicity. Sometimes referred to as "situational ethnicity," this assumption already has a place in the literature. The utilization of this assumption allows a focus on change, rather than a narrow focus on supposedly unvarying ethnic cultures.

The change process occurs within the ethnic group as it comes into contact with its host society. Both the structure of the group and the values and norms held by its individual members are altered. These alterations can result from a large number of factors, including the receptivity of the host society to the ethnic group, the economic and social opportunities for the ethnic group, its age configuration and needs, and the similarity or differences in values between the host society and ethnic group. As these variables are examined, it becomes clear that the effects of person–environment contact are not necessarily the same for the ethnic aged as for younger persons. The effects may also be different for first-generation immigrants than for third- or fourth-generation Americans.

The current paradigmatic approach to research on the ethnic aged needs to be reexamined to ensure that it does not lead research and practice into approaches that are not only misleading, but also conceivably harmful. Unfortunately, that is not the end of the process. New assumptions will only accurately describe the situation of the ethnic aged for a short time, and consequently the assumptions upon which research and planning are based will require a recurring cycle of re-examination. The result is that social scientists must view the world of the ethnic aged as one that is always emergent.

ASSESSING ETHNICITY

Beyond creation of a greater understanding of the relationship between aging and ethnicity service, providers need assistance in assessing the importance of ethnic background to an individual older person. Based on the discussion in the previous chapter, it is possible to develop a model that can be utilized for this purpose (Figure 8.1). The model brings together many of the issues discussed in earlier chapters.

Ethnic Background

The first element in the figure is the divergent ethnic cultures that exist in the United States. The terms *Black, Latino, Native American, Asian,* and *White* are relevant terms in this country. Beyond the ability of these terms to help individuals categorize others, they are important administratively in the designation of minorities for programs. As diver-

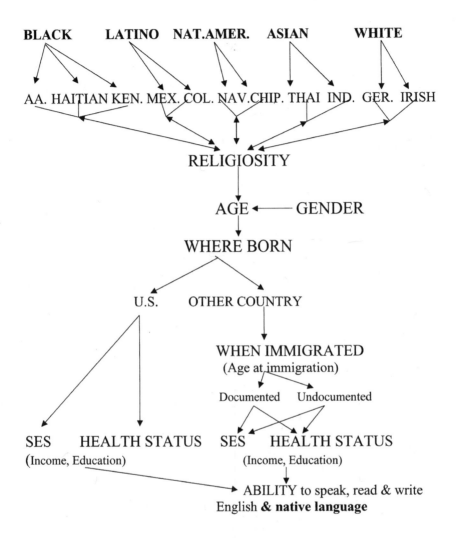

FIGURE 8.1 **Factors in providing services to the ethnic aged.**

sity has increased in the United States, larger numbers of groups have come to be lumped under these designations.

Older persons who are designated as Black in a local community may be Haitian or from an African country, as well as African American. Latinos in the United States include individuals from a large number of South and Central American countries, including Mexico and Columbia. Although there are commonalities among Native American cultures, western tribes, such as Navajos, are quick to point out the differences in their culture from eastern tribes, such as Chippewas. Even neighboring tribes, such as Hopis and Navajos, are distinctly different in language and many cultural attributes. Asian cultures, such as Thai or Indian, share some characteristics, but a lack of understanding among providers of important historical conflicts among many Asian groups, such as Japanese and Koreans, can damage their efforts to develop programs and services for these populations. Arab populations in the United States became a focus of attention after the tragedy of September 11, 2001, but, clearly, many Americans did not understand the diversity within this population. As well as being from a variety of different countries, there are Arabs whose religious affiliations are Christian and Muslim and Jewish.

Age

Providers, considering how and what services an older person from a particular ethnic background needs, must differentiate between the effects of chronological age and age cohort. Chronological age may partially explain the chronic health conditions affecting a client. The fact that, when they were young, adequate health care was not available to individuals in their ethnic group, or to lower-income individuals, may also explain why they have some chronic health problems not present among other individuals of the same age. Period effects related to an age cohort may also explain why some older individuals have limited reading ability. This understanding helps avoid the mistaken belief that lower reading scores among some older people is an indication of limited or declining intelligence.

Gender

Besides differences in life expectancy, the social aspects of aging appear to be different for men and women in most cultures. Roles for women may vary at all ages, but caregiving roles appear to be predominantly occupied by women.

Because of cultural norms regarding work outside the home, as well as discrimination, the economic resources many women have when they enter their later years are often dramatically lower than those of men. In the United States, women have lower salaries than men and may be employed in jobs in which they are not covered by Social Security. As a consequence, women, on average, have lower Social Security benefits than men. These lower benefits affect the ability of women from many ethnic groups to live adequately in the community.

Psychologically, women may view growing older differently than men and utilize different coping strategies to confront changes in their social status, roles, or health conditions. The social support mechanisms mobilized by women in many ethnic groups may differ from those called upon by men.

Spirituality and Religiosity

Religion and many ethnic cultures are strongly intertwined. This may be most true of cultures that are strongly Muslim in background, but it is also true of many ethnic groups that are primarily Catholic in religious orientation. Even in these cases, religious identity and religious practice can vary. Catholicism, as it developed in Ireland, France, Italy, or Poland, has many differences. Catholicism in Central and South America, or among Native Americans, may be combined with many elements of indigenous religious beliefs. Among Muslims, the differences between Sunnis and Shiites have created animosities visible in the war between Iran and Iraq in the 1990s.

Chapter 5 emphasizes the importance of separating religious institutions from religiosity. It is also important to recognize that spirituality may be found among individuals who are not believers in any theology. Spirituality and religiosity may have an impact on how individuals view the process of growing older, and even what health care is appropriate for their conditions.

In Figure 8.1, the arrows between religiosity and the various ethnic cultures are shown as two-sided. Although this adds complexity to the figure, it indicates that the relationship between religiosity and ethnic cultures is also complex. Ethnic cultures may influence religious beliefs and practices, but religious values may also influence the ethnic values of many groups. At times, separating these two elements may be difficult, for example, when maintaining that the roles allowed or not allowed for Iranian women are elements of Iranian culture and not related to Muslim religious beliefs as they are interpreted in Iran.

Personal History

Accurate assessment of an individual's needs requires avoidance of ethnic stereotypes. As already noted, providers who complete limited training about cultural diversity may use their knowledge about the culture of a client to assume behavior and attitudes of a particular individual. By not asking important questions of the client, the provider may make important and mistaken assumptions about the client.

Among the most important facts that a provider needs to ascertain is where the client was born. An older Chinese woman born in China may approach many aspects of life differently than an older Chinese woman born in the United States. The older Chinese woman born in China may have attitudes reflective of traditional Chinese culture; the older Chinese woman born in California or New York may differ dramatically in their norms and values. The degree of change or acculturation may also be related to the older woman's cohort of immigration. Grandchildren of Chinese laborers who built the American railroads may exhibit different attitudes than children of immigrants. Erdmans (1995) illustrates how individuals from the same ethnic background, living in the same community, can view their ethnic culture differently. In her discussion of Poles in Chicago, she differentiates between individuals who are new immigrants to the area (immigrants) and individuals who are from a Polish background (ethnics).

Understanding immigrants requires not only an understanding of the age of individuals in this population, but also such factors as the age when they emigrated. The life course of individuals who emigrate from a foreign country when they are young is potentially very different than the life course of individuals who arrive in the United States when they are 70 years old. The young person has the opportunity to obtain an education that ensures economic and social mobility. This education includes fluency in English, which is often difficult for older individuals to attain. The younger individual, interacting with individuals from other ethnic cultures, is exposed to cultural beliefs and responses to situations that differ from their own. Over time, these interaction patterns may result in changes in their own thinking and acculturation to norms that are considered American. This acculturation does not mean that the person completely abandons their culture. As discussed, individuals may range in their degree of acculturation, from adhering fully to traditional norms and values to complete assimilation into the culture of their new country.

Immigration Status

Despite the fact that many immigration advocates argue that national borders are artificial, restrictions are placed on from which countries immigrants will be accepted into the United States, and eligibility for programs once immigrants are admitted. Undocumented immigrants are officially ineligible for many programs. Fear of deportation may deter them from applying for many programs, even if these programs do not inquire about immigration status.

Often overlooked in the discussion of immigration status is the fact that undocumented immigrants are not likely to interact with individuals outside their ethnic group. The impact of this lack of interethnic contact can be substantial. One possible impact is limited knowledge of programs and services available in the community. Restrictions of interaction to individuals from the same background may also retard the ability of immigrants to find or obtain high-wage jobs.

Socioeconomic Status

The impact of socioeconomic status (income, education) on the ethnic aged has already been remarked upon. What is important is to recognize that socioeconomic diversity has increased among the ethnic aged, and will probably continue to increase. This means that the opportunities for education and reductions in discrimination have resulted in individuals from many ethnic groups obtaining higher incomes during their working years. The result is a growing group of ethnic aged with private pensions and other assets to supplement their income. Unfortunately, the disparity in these assets between Whites and Latinos, African Americans, and Native Americans is still dramatic. Positive economic conditions in the United States during the twenty-first century would help to ensure that each succeeding cohort of ethnic aged has a higher socioeconomic status than their predecessors.

Overall positive socioeconomic change among the ethnic aged is dependent to some extent on the number and background of immigrants who enter the country. If men and women from highly educated, professional backgrounds, such as those from India, continue to enter the country, it is easy to predict that they will be a group of ethnic aged with many resources to meet their needs. Immigrants from India with minimal education and training will be an older population with more extensive needs for social and health services.

Socioeconomic status is not only a matter of the economic resources of the older person. The higher socioeconomic status individual with a college degree may have extensive knowledge about health conditions. They may read material about preventive health care that they can undertake. They may also know what social services are available to assist them. Lacking this knowledge, they may not know how to obtain the needed information. Having learned whether they are eligible for these services, individuals with more education will not be fazed by the complex forms that are often required to obtain social or health services.

Language Fluency

Older people vary in their language fluency. Ethnic aged, who came to the United States from another country at a young age, may be able to read and write English as well as their native language. However, some of these immigrants may have obtained only limited education in their own country. The result is that they enter the country unable to read and write in their native tongue. If they have opportunities for education in the country, then they may become fluent in English, without ever being able to read or write the language of their homeland. Individuals who emigrate when they are middle-aged or older may have the dual problem of never having received adequate education in their homeland or in the United States.

Varied levels of speaking, reading, and writing English and a native tongue have an impact on efforts to disseminate information and promote a variety of health and social service programs for older persons. Because of literacy problems, materials developed for the ethnic aged must be carefully designed to accommodate these low levels of literacy (Sabogal, Otero-Sabogal, Pasick, Jenkins, & Perez-Stable, 1996). Careful development of these materials requires a knowledge of the possibility that not only does the older person have only limited literacy in English, but also perhaps in their native tongue.

THE FUTURE OF ETHNICITY AND AGING

Social science always attempts to explain a changing reality. The society that could identify the values and occupational and educational characteristics of ethnic groups without hesitation, in 1900, now has to employ many qualifiers to discuss the Italians, Jews, African Americans, and Japanese of the twenty-first century. The qualifiers represent disparate educational and income levels among these populations. In the twenty-first century, ethnicity will not have the same salience for all groups. Alba's (1990) analysis of data, collected among individuals from various European ethnic groups living in the Albany region of New York, indicates that ethnic identities are becoming less important among these groups. This attenuated identity is evidenced by intermarriage patterns, language use, and culturally specific allegiances. A generalized European identity remains important to these individuals, rather than identification with being Irish, Italian, and so on.

Historically, the trend around the world has been to submerge ethnic identity under a national identity. In Spain, Basques from northern Spain were expected to accept their place as Spaniards. Aboriginals in Australia were expected to accept Australian identity. Rival tribal groups in Somalia and Rwanda were expected to overcome their long-standing differences for the sake of their new country. In Yugoslavia, Croat, Bosnians, and Serbs were expected to learn tolerance for each other in the country founded after World War I. In the United States, Native Americans were expected to appreciate American citizenship and lessen their identity with tribal cultures.

These expectations have not been met. Native American cultures are now resurgent and exerting political power. Yugoslavia has been cleaved into individual parts as a result of interethnic conflicts. In Rwanda, ethnic conflicts in the 1990s resulted in massive slaughter of Tutsis by Hutus. In Somalia, rivalries between tribal groups have resulted in warfare and a nonfunctioning central government. In Spain, a separatist Basque movement continues violence and bombings.

Poor economic conditions and political repression continue to encourage immigration around the world. The United States focuses on immigration from Latin America and Asia, Italy is concerned about immigrants from Albania, Spain and France about North Africans, England about Caribbeans and Asians, and Germany about immigrants from a variety of countries.

Immigrants in some countries were originally invited or brought in to provide laborers. The use of slaves in the United States and the Caribbean enabled large cotton and sugar plantations in these two areas. In Germany, a shortage of workers after World War II resulted in the government instituting a program of "guest workers." A similar program in the United States enabled growers to bring in Mexican laborers to pick crops.

These controlled immigrations are now a remnant of the past. Undocumented workers and asylum seekers continue to arrive in small boats, walk across deserts, and stow away in cargo containers on trucks, in efforts to leave their home countries. Individuals entering the United States on tourist visas remain after the visas expire, and try to blend into the general population. In Germany, guest workers who came from Turkey and Greece have stayed and raised children in their new country.

With immigration at a high point around the world, complaints about individuals from different ethnic backgrounds have taken on a similar tone in different countries. The complaints usually stress that immigrants take away jobs from natives, immigrants are willing to work for low wages and reduce salaries for native workers, immigrants commit crimes, and immigrants are unwilling to acculturate and insist on only living and associating with "their own." These complaints are similar to complaints about immigrants in earlier periods of history, but the ubiquity of immigrants throughout developed countries magnifies their visibility.

The responses that will be made to these complaints by citizens of different countries remains to be seen, but these responses will affect the socioeconomic and political status of the ethnic aged. At this point, no definitive portrayal of the future role of ethnicity among the aged in the United States can be provided. It is possible, however, to discern some of the factors that will play an important role in the meaning of ethnicity for aging during the next century. These include immigration policies, fertility, marriage patterns, intermarriage, and attitudes toward multiculturalism.

Immigration Policies

There are indications that United States immigration policies are shifting away from those that favor family preference, to a point-type system. Under this system, applicants for immigration will be given preference on the basis of the number of points they accumulate. More points may be given to individuals under age 45 with higher educational backgrounds than to older or less-educated individuals. A system of this type already exists in other countries.

Because of higher educational levels, but less recent arrival of family members in the United States, a point system will increase the opportunity for individuals from European countries to immigrate. It will probably reduce the number of immigrants from Latin America. Other options that have already been adopted in this country include placing more emphasis on preferences related to occupations, earmarking a portion of total immigration quotas for individuals from a certain country, and adoption of a lottery system for countries underrepresented in current immigration figures. None of these changes will fundamentally alter the flow of undocumented immigrants from Latin America, or even China, to the United States. Unless effective mechanisms of enforcement are found, or economic and political conditions improve in their home countries, undocumented immigrants will continue to be the largest component of America's new immigrants.

Fertility

Total fertility rates in the United States are expected to decline from their current levels. Declines were also expected to occur among ethnic groups with high fertility rates. This expectation has not been met. Childbearing rates for African American and Latino women still remain high. High fertility rates have both positive and negative impacts. From the perspective of the older person, it may appear that a larger number of children means that more individuals will be available to provide them with assistance as they grow older. High fertility rates, however, also mean that there are more stresses placed on potential caregivers who are faced not only with assistance to older parents but also to young children. A recent study (American Association of Retired Persons, n.d.) indicates that women between the ages of 45 and 55 are primary providers of assistance to older relatives. These women in the middle often feel they are not providing adequate assistance, and express guilt about the amount of care they are able to provide. This sense of guilt was found among all groups, but was strongest among Asians.

Marriage Patterns

There has clearly been a trend toward later first marriage among women in the United States. Equally important is the number of people who never marry. The never-married group has accounted for about 5% of the population for many years, but there are increasing numbers of never-married individuals in the country. This group is larger among African Americans than among Whites. In 1990, 75% of Black women ages 35–39 were married, compared to 91% of White women (Bovee, 1992). Thus, this group of Black women will probably have a higher proportion of unmarried individuals when they reach the ages of 50 and 60.

In contemporary America, "singlehood" does not mean that women do not have children or long-term relationships with men. Many of these never-married African American women may take on traditional caregiving roles and receive assistance from adult children when they age. Without these male partners and adult children, however, never-married older African American women will have to rely on other informal and formal sources of support. Increased proportions of never-married individuals among other ethnic groups will have the same impact, increasing the demands on a variety of social service organizations.

Intermarriage

As intermarriage occurs, the likelihood of important value shifts increases. Intermarriage rates between two distinct ethnic cultures cannot reveal the process of cultural change that takes place within a couple. Does one culture become predominant, and what is the basis of that predominance? Is there a symbiosis of cultures, with an emergent cultural pattern, which is, for example, neither Irish nor Italian, but maintains elements of both ethnic cultures? Is there an abandonment of any overt allegiance to ethnic culture, and a conscious decision that children should be brought up only as "Americans?" Decision-making by an intermarried couple may not be as clear-cut as these questions would imply. As Jarvempa (1985) remarks about intermarriage among Native Americans, the "non-Indian partner experiences resocialization into an Indian subsociety" (p. 37). This resocialization can result in internalization of Indian norms and rearing of children with strong values of the Native American tribe. Intermarriage by Latinos raises similar questions. According to one estimate, by 2050, more than 40% of Latinos in the United States will be from multiple ethnic backgrounds (Smith, cited in Rodriguez, 2001).

Attitudes About Multiculturalism

A society experiencing a growth of ethnic populations may adopt a number of responses toward these groups. One possibility is adoption of an overt pluralistic model, as in Australia's current multicultural policy. In this model, differing behaviors and differing approaches to meeting common needs are seen as equally valid. On the other hand, the host environment may view any deviation from the majority's attitudes and behaviors as negative.

In a pluralistic society, the majority will also support varied approaches to aging among ethnic groups, including distinctive methods utilized to provide assistance to older persons. In a less tolerant society, African Americans, Latinos, Asians, Native Americans, and White ethnic groups have to alter their assistance patterns. They are required to utilize programs and service formats they may regard as inappropriate to their culture.

Ethnic groups can develop and operate their own programs and services. This tactic was characteristic of many earlier European immigrant groups in the United States. The 2000 census indicates that there will be no lack of ethnic populations to serve during the next century. Presently, lacking among many of these currently underserved groups are the socioeconomic resources necessary to develop their own programs.

Sufficient socioeconomic resources allow decisions about adherence to traditional ethnic norms to be based on preference rather than necessity. An example of this preference can be found among Japanese Americans: "The Issei (first-generation immigrants) cling to tradition, the Nisei (second generation) shy away from it, and the Sansei (third generation)—despite their extensive acculturation—rediscover it. For the Issei, tradition is a way of life, but for the Sansei it is an object of intellectual curiosity and a search for identity" (Osako & Liu, 1986). The Sansei possess higher socioeconomic status than their grandparents. The opportunities for education and higher-level jobs are thus key elements in increasing the options of ethnic families. Having these options may result in a deviation by family members from traditional approaches to aging. This could include models of family assistance, since both sons and daughters may be employed outside the home. This deviation, however, will be based on decisions about what is most valued, rather than mere survival.

Economic Structures and the Ethnic Aged

The poor ethnic aged face many challenges in their later years. The problems facing these ethnic aged stem from the lack of opportunities or from discrimination they encountered at earlier points in their lives. The issue confronting the United States is how to ensure that the numbers of poor ethnic aged in the twenty-first century is limited.

Economic opportunities for young people are needed, so that, as they move into their later years, they will have the socioeconomic resources they require. Taking advantage of the best economic opportunities in modern America requires a college education. During most of the twentieth century, men and women who did not have college degrees were still able to obtain adequate income from the many manufacturing jobs throughout the country. Even facing major discrimination, many African Americans and Latinos were able to find work in some manufacturing sectors, such as the automobile industry. Technological changes, and the shifting of jobs by multinational corporations to lower-wage, developing countries, have reduced the availability of these jobs. Service jobs in hotels and fast food restaurants will not meet the economic needs of people as they grow older.

The needs of the ethnic aged in the United States cannot be separated from the needs of their larger group and the changes taking place in American society. The extent of the American commitment to meeting the needs of its residents of all ages will determine the future status of the ethnic aged.

REFERENCES

American Association of Retired Persons (AARP). (n.d.). *In the middle.* Retrieved May 20, 2002, from *http://research.aarp.org/il/in_the_middle.html*

Alba, R. (1990). *Ethnic identity: The transformation of White America.* New Haven, CT: Yale University Press.

Bovee, T. (1992, March 4). Marriage rate lower for black women. *Detroit Free Press,* 3A.

Erdmans, M. (1995). Immigrants and ethnics: Conflict and identity in Chicago Polonia. *Sociological Quarterly, 36,* 175–195.

Jarvempa, R. (1985). The political economy and political ethnicity of American Indian adaptations and identities. In R. Alba (Ed.), *Ethnicity and race in the U.S.A.: Towards the 21st century* (pp. 29–48). Boston: Routledge and Kegan Paul.

Kitano, H. (1969). *Japanese Americans.* Englewood Cliffs, NJ: Prentice-Hall.

Kuhn, T. (1962). *The structure of scientific revolutions.* Chicago: University of Chicago Press.

Nelson, E., & Dannefer, D. (1992). Aged heterogeneity: Fact or fiction? The fate of diversity in gerontological research. *The Gerontologist, 32,* 17–23.

Nydegger, C. (1983). Family ties of the aged in cross-cultural perspective. *The Gerontologist, 23,* 26–32.

Osako, M., & Liu, W. (1986). Intergenerational relationships and the aged among Japanese Americans. *Research on Aging, 8,* 128–155.

Rodriguez, G. (2001, February 11). Mexican-Americans: Forging a new vision of America's melting pot. *New York Times,* pp. 4:1, 4.

Sabogal, F., Otero-Sabogal, R., Pasick, R., Jenkins, C., & Perez-Stable, E. (1996). Printed health education materials for diverse communities: Suggestions learned from the field. *Health Education Quarterly, 23*(Suppl.), S123–141.

U.S. Census Bureau. (2001). *Profile of general demographic characteristics: 2000.* Retrieved June 22, 2002, from *http://www.factfinder.census/gov*

Index